Best Supplements for Men

For More Muscle, Higher Testosterone, Longer Life,
and Better Looks

P. D. Mangan

Best Supplements for Men.

Disclaimer

This book contains general information about medical conditions and treatments. The author is not a physician or healthcare practitioner, and the information in this book is not advice and should not be treated as such.

The information in this book is provided "as is" without any representations or warranties, express or implied.

Without prejudice to the generality of the foregoing paragraph, the author does not warrant that:

The information in this book will be constantly available, or available at all;

The medical information in this book is complete, true, accurate, up-to-date, or non-misleading.

You must not rely on the information in this book as an alternative to medical advice from your doctor or other professional healthcare provider.

If you have any specific questions about any medical matter you should consult your doctor or other professional healthcare provider.

If you think you may be suffering from any medical condition you should seek immediate medical attention.

You should never delay seeking medical advice, disregard medical advice, or discontinue medical treatment because of information in this book.

You should consult your doctor or other professional healthcare provider before undertaking any diet or exercise program, or taking any vitamin, mineral, or other supplement.

Nothing in this medical disclaimer will limit any of our liabilities in any way that is not permitted under applicable law, or exclude any of our liabilities that may not be excluded under applicable law.

CONTENTS

1: Why Supplements?

Supplements are over-the-counter (no prescription needed) substances that contain concentrated amounts of nutrients or other substances that can benefit health.

The question naturally arises, do we need supplements? If we're in decent health and don't suffer from any obvious nutritional deficiencies, aren't supplements superfluous? Many skeptics, most of whom seem to be doctors, talk of supplements merely as a means of making "expensive urine", the idea being that we spend a lot of money on them, they don't do anything much, and we excrete them in our urine, a waste in more than one sense of the word.

The idea of "expensive urine" does have some merit. Many of the supplements that are marketed and sold are simply not necessary, and one of the main objects of this book is to show which supplements you don't need and are a waste of money, and which ones can improve your health.

Mangan's Rule of Supplements

Which supplements aren't necessary? A consideration of that question and of what unnecessary supplements have in common led me to formulate Mangan's Rule of Supplements:

The higher priced the supplement, the less likely you are to benefit from it.

Most beneficial supplements that I discuss in this book are inexpensive, because the basic substances that confer health benefits are all unpatented and generic. More expensive supplements may be proprietary blends of cheaper ones, so that you end up paying extra for some alleged knowledge of the correct proportion of ingredients. Or they may prey on the consumer's ignorance, who doesn't know that the supplement in question should be cheap.

Pre-workout supplements are good examples of unnecessary and/or expensive supplements. Most of them are blends of caffeine and protein, and promise better performance in the gym, but you can easily duplicate them and much more cheaply by drinking coffee and using whey protein. When they contain ingredients other than caffeine or protein, they often don't work well or could be harmful.

Some anti-aging supplements on the market may also fit this bill. My favorite example is nicotinamide riboside (NR), which is both expensive and touted as a uniquely powerful anti-aging molecule. But the first half of this substance is nicotinamide, and that's merely a form of vitamin B3, which is not only cheap but appears to raise NAD+ levels, the anti-aging target, as much as the more expensive riboside form. Time will tell whether NR reaches its potential and is actually more effective than plain old vitamin B3, but for now, I advise people to stay away from a product that costs $50 a month and isn't proven to be better than a cheap product.

I'll also show you how to make cheap anti-aging supplements, cutting the cost of some of the proprietary blends way down from the $30 to $50 a month they charge for them.

Raspberry ketones are another useless supplement: they don't cause weight loss and they're expensive. I suspect that marketers prey on people's vague sense that "ketones" are beneficial – and they are – but pull the old switcheroo and sell them something that just sounds similar.

One thing I'll do in this book is provide the reader with guidance on which supplements are beneficial and in what cases. I won't mention all the supplements that I think overpriced or of little use, but if it isn't listed here, that's probably the case.

But on to why we might need supplements.

1. We don't always eat right

Many of us do not always eat what's best for us, and supplements can make a difference in our health.

A recent report found that Americans eat close to 60% of their calories as ultra-processed foods and added sugars.[1] That's part of what led to the obesity disaster that the U.S. (and increasingly the rest of the world) faces. Eating such a huge amount of ultra-processed food and sugar can leave us open to nutritional deficiencies, and supplements may go some way toward correcting them. While supplements can't completely mitigate the harm to eating processed food, they can help – although my first piece of advice would be to quit eating all that garbage and to eat whole, minimally-processed food.

Even if we do eat right, many of our foods don't contain sufficient or optimal amounts of nutrients. They may be grown on soil that's been depleted of essential minerals. Or they may be raised in conditions that don't leave optimal nutrients in the food; farm-raised salmon, for example, in contrast to wild salmon, contains low amounts of the important omega-3 fatty acids; grain-fed chicken contain high amounts of omega-6 fatty acids. Supplements can help in these cases. The war on

6

saturated fat has taken a toll on eating meat, with subsequent non-optimal intake of essential minerals like zinc.

We don't always drink right either. Hard water used to be a significant source of magnesium in our diets, but hardly anyone drinks it anymore and many if not most people in the modern, developed world are magnesium deficient.

2. Poor lifestyles

Many of us burn the candle at both ends, don't sleep well enough, are cooped up in office cubicles all day long, sometimes drink more alcohol than is good for us, and commit other sins against a healthy life. (Hey, it ain't easy being a saint all the time.)

Supplements can help correct some of our lifestyle excesses and defects. For instance, if you don't get any sunshine, and I mean full-body exposure for 20 minutes (at least) daily, and at a lower latitude in summer, you could be vitamin D deficient. Vitamin D supplements can help to compensate for your lifestyle, where you live, and the season of the year.

If you have trouble sleeping because of shift work, stress, or for any other reason, melatonin could help you sleep and make you healthier and even live longer.

Whey protein could give you a quick protein boost when you don't have enough time to make a proper meal, and add to your daily protein intake such that you reach an optimal amount for muscle growth. Some supplements may even give you some of the same benefits as exercise.

There are many other examples, which we'll discuss. The right supplements can get you healthier.

3. Fighting aging

Many of the supplements we'll discuss help fight the aging process.

Let's be clear: aging is entirely natural. Nature and evolution don't care if you die of old age; nature's purpose is for you to have lots of children, or die trying. (Maybe *and* die trying.) To fight aging, you must fight nature to an extent.

While most of the anti-aging supplements in this book are natural and not synthetic chemical substances (which are drugs), they are usually found in small quantities in natural products, so to make use of them, concentrated versions, or supplements, may be indicated. For example, red wine contains the anti-aging compound resveratrol, but to get a useful amount of resveratrol from wine, you'd have to drink around 50 bottles a day. Impossible, and highly undesirable. Berberine, another anti-aging compound, comes from traditional Chinese medicine, and it's impossible to get enough from food or other herbal sources.

4. Decent versus optimal health

If you have decent health and are satisfied with it, and are satisfied with the average life expectancy for an American man (about 79 years), then don't worry about supplements.

But if you want to take your health to the next level, supplements can help you to do so. You could be lifting weights and fathering children long after your compatriots have met the Grim Reaper, if you do it right.

5. Optimal body composition and weight loss

Some supplements can boost your weight loss and your muscle-gaining efforts. Berberine, for instance, functions similarly to the prescription anti-diabetic drug metformin, and fat loss, along with improved insulin sensitivity (a very good thing), are two of the benefits of berberine.

Whey protein is an essential supplement for the strength trainer, and can help build more muscle when taken immediately before or after a session of lifting weights.

Vitamin D deficiency is associated with obesity. The list goes on.

6. Testosterone

The men of the U.S. and Europe are facing a long-term decline in testosterone, the hormone that makes men manly. Not only do men have lower testosterone levels as they age, but at the same age now, as opposed to a few decades ago, a man has lower testosterone. In other words, a 40-year-old man now has lower testosterone than a 40-year-old man did 30 years ago. The causes are still being debated, and no clear consensus has emerged.

Certain supplements can help boost testosterone. Not only do these supplements do that, but using other supplements, such as vitamin D, magnesium, and zinc, that keep your entire body finely tuned, can increase your testosterone.

You're not going to increase testosterone levels on a standard American diet, that's for sure, and that diet will likely decrease them.

You can't outrun a bad diet

There's an expression about exercise to the effect that you can't outrun a bad diet, meaning that no amount of exercise can help with weight loss if you don't eat properly.

While supplements can help, I want to emphasize that should you decide to use them, you should also concentrate on other important lifestyle factors, such as diet. And sleep. Exercise. Keeping stress and anxiety at bay.

All of these are important, arguably more important than many supplements, unless perhaps you suffer from a serious nutritional deficiency.

So, don't eat processed food if you can help it. Avoid sugar, flour, and vegetable oils (not including olive oil.) Sleep 7 to 8 hours a night. Get some sunshine. Don't stress out. Lift weights, do some high-intensity interval training. (My preferred forms of exercise, and arguably the best.)

Supplements are cheaper than drugs and in some cases more effective

We're living in an era with doctors prescribing from a seemingly endless arsenal of drugs. While doctors get some criticism for doing that, the reality is that most people would rather take pills than do anything about changing their lifestyles.

Pharmaceutical companies also promote drugs, and it's no wonder, as they can be expensive. The money factor in modern medicine is huge; older treatments often don't give way to new and better ones because there's less money in the newer ones. By the same token, newer drugs get introduced precisely because they're highly profitable.

Many drugs have supplement counterparts that can do the same job at a cheaper price and don't require a prescription. Take berberine, for example. This supplement lowers blood sugar in diabetics as well as its counterpart metformin, a prescription drug. If you're suffering from anxiety, the inexpensive supplement theanine relieves anxiety without the dangerous side effects of prescription anxiolytics (tranquilizers), and can improve your health while doing so; anxiolytics and antidepressants generally have a terrible safety record and may kill millions of people in the U.S. and Europe annually.[2]

Omega-3 fatty acids (from fish oil) may prevent heart attacks better than any prescription statin drug, and curcumin, green tea, and IP6 prevent cancer better than any prescription drug. (The only drugs shown to prevent cancer are metformin, noted above, and rapamycin, an immunosuppressant not available to anyone but transplant patients.)

Aspirin, assuredly not a supplement but a cheap over-the-counter drug, extends life (in lab animals), decreases cancer and heart attacks (in humans), and is an underutilized medicine for which no real prescription counterpart exists.

In short, the right supplements may keep you healthier than an expensive prescription drug with lots of side effects, and you don't even have to see your doctor for a prescription, nor a pharmacy to obtain them. Your doctor won't be telling you about all this, I can all but guarantee it. Most doctors simply don't know anything about them, care less, and have little incentive to instruct their patients in their use, assuming they know how in the first place.

Plan of the book

I haven't listed every single supplement one could possibly use, which would in any case be an impossible task.

The supplements that I've written about are those that seem to me to have the best evidence for efficacy and safety.

I've grouped supplements according to their major uses or effects, but many of them have major effects in more than one category. That's to be expected, since anything that improves overall health improves the function of any single aspect of health. For example, a man in good health ought to have a normal testosterone level, so something that improves a man's health will optimize his testosterone.

2: Muscle, Strength, and Energy

Muscle is a very underrated factor in health and lifespan. More muscle means better health and longer life, better metabolism, and greater insulin sensitivity.[1]

Muscle isn't free, however, and while young people at the age of maturity, around 20 years of age, may have lots of muscle, as you age you increasingly have to work for it. Without the necessary work, the average man (and woman) loses about 10% of their muscle with each passing decade, and by the time a man is 80, he will on average have lost half of his muscle mass. It's not a coincidence that the average man's lifespan in the U.S. is about 80.

When muscle loss continues long enough, a condition known as sarcopenia results, which is muscle wasting. Sarcopenia causes frailty and dependence and often leads to life in a nursing home.

Even at younger ages, muscle loss leads to obesity and diabetes, since muscle acts as a metabolic "sink" that takes up blood sugar and acts to keep the entire body insulin sensitive. Regular exercise, although healthy, has a poor record at fat loss; exercise that adds muscle, strength training, has a much better record, since adding muscle increases fat-burning activity around the clock.

More muscle requires two things

Adding more muscle requires two things: 1) strength training and 2) protein. Strength training, such as weightlifting and other resistance training exercise such as bodyweight training, is the most potent stimulus for adding muscle, but to get the most out of them, you must consume an adequate amount of protein, which is at least 1.2 to 1.4 grams of protein per kilogram of bodyweight daily. (That's about 0.55 grams per pound of bodyweight.) A recent study using the indicator amino acid method (different from nitrogen balance) found that young male bodybuilders required an average of 1.7 g/kg of protein daily, so the question of the right amount of protein for muscle gains is actually still controversial.[2] Bodybuilders may actually require less protein than endurance athletes: most studies have shown that bodybuilders and strength trainers need a maximum of 1.8 g/kg.[3]

Protein supplements

Protein supplements are a good way to ensure that you get enough protein. By adding 20 grams or more of protein daily, in the form of a supplement, you can ensure you reach your daily protein goal, depending on your body weight and goals.

Perhaps more important, drinking a protein supplement immediately before or after a strength training workout boosts the process of muscle growth even more, so if you want to make the most of your training, a protein supplement is a must. Endurance athletes such as runners actually need more protein than strength athletes, so even if the goal of your sport or training isn't muscle growth, taking extra protein makes sense.

Protein supplements can boost muscle growth after a workout for a couple of different reasons. One is that the right supplement is *fast* protein, that is, it digests and is absorbed from the gut quickly. Immediately after a workout, muscles are primed for growth, but can't grow unless amino acids from protein are available; a fast protein allows the muscle to get immediate access to the necessary amino acids.

The second reason a protein supplement can boost muscle growth is its amino acid content. Protein is made of amino acids strung together. There are 20 different amino acids, and of these, the most important are the 9 so-called essential amino acids. They're essential because the human body can't make them and they must be ingested in the diet. Only the essential amino acids can increase muscle growth.

Branched-chain amino acids, leucine, and whey

Among the essential amino acids, a group of 3 stand out, and these are the branched-chain amino acids, or BCAAs: leucine, isoleucine, and valine. They act as signals for muscle growth. BCAAs from protein are the single most important factor in the nutritional promotion of muscle growth. Among the BCAAs, it's now understood that leucine is by far the most important molecule that signals muscles to grow.[4]

To grow muscle tissue optimally after a workout, consume protein with a high content of essential amino acids and BCAAs. The ideal protein that fits the bill is whey protein.

Whey protein is that fraction of milk that remains liquid when milk is curdled, and is the most popular protein supplement among bodybuilders and other strength athletes. Whey is about 50% essential amino acids, and about 25% BCAAs, with a leucine content of about 15%.[5] That makes whey ideal for post-workout protein.

Whey protein, with a high leucine content, can also help with fat loss. In overweight people, leucine at 2.25 grams, along with 30 mg of vitamin B6, taken 3 times daily, increased fat burning (oxidation) by about 50%.[6] That can really add up over time and result in significant fat loss. (But you still need to pay attention to diet and exercise.) Furthermore, adding whey protein to a weight-loss diet results in significantly more fat loss, almost double, and less muscle loss, about half, than those who didn't use whey.[7] The dose was 10 grams before breakfast and 10 before dinner.

Recovery

Recovery from exercise is an important but neglected concept, all the more important in strength training. When you put muscles through intense training as in weightlifting, they need time to recover, as long as 6 days until strength has recovered fully. Muscle grow outside the gym, not inside.

Before muscles have fully recovered, exercising them intensely could be counterproductive; speeding muscle recovery can ensure the ability to get back into the gym and train again. Whey protein can help recovery by supplying muscle with the right mix of essential and branched-chain amino acids.[8] Because of the effect on recovery, whey protein immediately after a strength-training workout can help you even if you eat adequate high-quality protein at your regular meals.

Anabolic Resistance

A fraction of muscle tissue breaks down and builds up every day, and this is a normal and healthy process. Fasting, such as overnight between dinner and breakfast, results in an increase in the breakdown of muscle tissue, and when we eat again, the tissue rebuilds.

When we're young, taking protein in a meal robustly increases the rate of muscle protein synthesis, resulting in a balance between breakdown and buildup. But as we age, this process goes awry, and with a long-term imbalance between breakdown and synthesis, we lose muscle mass. One of the causes of this (along with less physical activity) is *anabolic resistance*, which is the failure of muscle tissue to respond properly to dietary protein with increased growth.

While exercise seems to have the same muscle-building effect on old as on young people, this is not the case with protein. But the good news is that older people can overcome their anabolic resistance by consuming a greater amount of leucine-rich protein at each meal.[9] Whey is the best protein for this purpose, since it contains high amounts of leucine and is a concentrated form of protein, so the right amounts of leucine and protein can be easily consumed in a low-calorie form.

Even the oldest people, into their 80s and above, can build solid muscle with a combination of strength training and protein supplementation.[10]

BCAAs have been shown to increase the lifespan of lab animals, mice in this case.[11] They do this by increasing the numbers of the cell's mitochondria, the powerhouses of the cell. Since declining numbers and decreasing quality of mitochondria are strongly associated with aging, BCAAs could prevent or even reverse this process.

Protein timing

When you consume whey for muscle growth may matter a lot. Or it may not. Let me explain.

Many studies have found that consuming whey protein either immediately before or immediately after a strength-training workout strongly promotes muscle growth, as opposed to taking it several hours before or after. Other studies have been more equivocal, and a lively debate has surrounded this issue.[12] It appears that the amount of protein regularly consumed at meals matters for the protein timing effect; if you consume adequate protein most of the time, and you don't workout while fasting, protein timing may not be critical.

But if you don't eat enough protein, or eat it a long time after workouts, or if you are older and have some degree of anabolic resistance, protein timing may matter a lot.

Because this matter of protein timing isn't settled, and because it's not difficult to consume 20 to 25 grams of protein after a workout, and because maximizing muscle growth is one of the main goals of strength training, taking whey protein immediately before or after a workout makes sense. (Whether before or after works better has also been the subject of debate, but in my estimation of the scientific literature, either appears to be fine, and newbie strength trainers may want to do both.)

Casein protein

The other fraction of milk protein that is not whey, and which makes up about 80% of the total protein, is casein. One of the chief differences between casein and whey is the speed of digestion; as opposed to whey, casein is a slow-digesting protein. Whether casein or whey is better for muscle growth has also been the subject of much debate.

As we've noted, immediately around (before or after) a workout, a fast-digesting protein like whey ramps of muscle synthesis quickly; strength training primes a muscle to grow, and the addition of protein completes the set-up, and muscles then grow. This effect is at its peak immediately after a workout, so a fast protein makes sense in that context.

In other contexts, casein can make sense. If consumed at bedtime, for example, slow-digesting casein allows for a steady supply of amino acids in the blood stream all night, and that can mean better muscle growth and better exercise recovery.[13] If someone were to eat no regular food other than a protein supplement after a workout, casein might make more sense there as well, since casein will sustain the flow of amino acids. That might be the case for someone trying to lose fat.

Casein, however, doesn't seem to have the anti-aging effect of whey, and since I make a point of eating a regular meal shortly after strength training, I prefer fast-digesting whey.

The studies pointing to casein as a better option than whey don't take into account that people normally eat other food, not just protein drinks. These studies show that while whey provides a fast spike of amino acids, that spike drops fairly quickly, in about a couple of hours. Casein provides a slow, steady release of amino acids for several hours; but so does a normal protein meal. Normally, at some point not long after a strength-training (or other exercise) session, you would eat a regular meal with adequate protein, which releases amino acids into the bloodstream over a time frame of several hours. Hence, slow-digesting casein is superfluous in that case.

Casein makes a good meal replacement drink for strength trainers who are trying to both cut fat and gain muscle; 25 grams of casein provides only about 100 calories (same as whey), and its slow-digesting nature will keep essential amino acids flowing into the bloodstream and to the muscles for several hours. When cutting (fat), keeping calories low and protein intake adequate allows the fat to come off without compromising muscle mass and strength. So, someone trying to cut fat while retaining muscle could take 25 grams of casein protein as a lunch substitute, for example.

Glutathione and cysteine

Whey contains a high amount of the amino acid cysteine, which is important for the synthesis of glutathione.

Glutathione is the centerpiece of the body's internal antioxidant system. No doubt you've heard that free radicals are bad and antioxidants are good, but that's a gross oversimplification. Some free radicals are bad, and some antioxidants are good. (We'll have more to say or antioxidants later.)

Free radicals are bad in excess, but they are aɪʃʊ important signaling molecules, so the body strives to keep their levels within a certain range, not too high or low. It uses its own antioxidants, including glutathione, to do this. When free radicals are generated in excess, such as in disease, aging, or even excessive exercise, glutathione is used up and the body enters a state called oxidative stress. To deal with oxidative stress, the body needs to make more glutathione from amino acids, and of these, cysteine is the most important, the rate-limiting step, i.e. no cysteine, no glutathione.

Replenishing glutathione by ensuring adequate intake of cysteine can alleviate oxidative stress and can therefore be important in improving health. It may be especially important in states of fatigue, as I discussed at length in my book, *Smash Chronic Fatigue*.

Whey is highest in cysteine of all proteins.

How to use whey protein

While whey protein robustly promotes muscle growth, you must consume enough of it at one time for it to work properly. For young people in good health, 20 grams suffices to potently stimulate muscle protein synthesis. For older people, up to 40 grams may be necessary.

- Either pre- or post-workout, take 20 grams of whey protein. Strength-training beginners, who pack on muscle faster than veteran trainers, may want to take 20 grams of whey both before and after training.

- To lose weight, suggested use is 10 grams before breakfast and 10 before dinner. Alternatively, 20 grams of whey used as a meal substitute. That will promote fat loss without muscle loss.
- To fight sarcopenia, one study of elderly people used 20 grams of whey at both breakfast and lunch, in addition to the normal diet.[14]

Suggested Protein Supplements

Protein supplements have become popular, and these days, hundreds, even thousands of protein supplements are on the market. Choosing the right one can be difficult. Generally, whey protein that is minimally processed is best. Some manufacturers use a heat- or chemical-based process to make whey protein, and these should be avoided if possible, although discovering how a particular product is made is not always easy. Look for non-denatured, cold-processed whey.

Among the best protein supplement brands are NutraBio, Bulk Supplements, and Optimum Nutrition, although there are many others.

Among the worst are Muscle Milk, which contains fructose and vegetable oils; mass gainers, which are extremely high in calories; ready-made protein drinks that contain soy and sugar; and protein bars, which usually have lots of sugar, industrial seed oils, and other junk ingredients.

Mass Gainers and Protein Bars

Mass gainers make a bad choice for weight gain; almost all of them contain loads of sugar, chemical ingredients, and industrial products that pass for food, such as vegetable oils.

Mass gainers usually contain a decent amount of protein, but they add a ton of carbohydrates for weight gain, as many as 250 grams in some products, total macronutrients adding up to 1200 calories or more a serving. While they may work for gaining weight, the kind of weight you gain isn't likely to be the kind you want: mostly fat, little muscle.

There's a limit to the rate at which you can gain muscle; you can't force the issue with mass gainers or indeed any other way. While dedicated strength training, adequate protein, and the right number of calories can build muscle optimally, simply pouring lots of calories into your system won't build muscle. Instead, the massive carbohydrates in mass gainers spike insulin, and all those calories end up as fat. The theory behind mass gainers is flawed, unless you count extra fat tissue as mass, but in that case, most people don't have much trouble with putting on fat mass. If all that isn't enough, mass gainers are expensive too.

Some men (and women) may have trouble getting enough calories from real food, but based on observational evidence – a combined 70% rate of overweight and obesity in the U.S. – that probably doesn't apply to many. But if you do want to gain weight and have difficulty doing so, a better option would be to make your own mass gainer from real food, not from industrial products and sugar. For example, here's a weight-gain shake recipe:

- 2 scoops whey protein
- 12 ounces whole milk
- 2 tablespoons almond butter
- 1 banana

Blend ingredients. Drink. It provides just over 700 calories and 65 grams of protein, with no added chemicals or industrial frankenfoods. Many more weight-gain shake recipes like this, using whole, natural ingredients, can be found on the internet.

Protein bars are basically just candy bars with some added protein. Like many of the mass gainers, they contain sugar and vegetable oils. Companies that make protein bars sometimes get around listing sugar in their ingredients by using dates as the sugar source, or sometimes fruit juice, but don't be fooled, that's sugar. A typical bestselling protein bar has 360 calories and 20 grams of protein, but a whopping 29 grams (about 6 teaspoons) of sugar.

If you need to grab some high-quality protein on the go, try hard-boiled eggs, which can be made by the dozen and stored in the fridge. Each one has about 8 grams of protein, 80 calories, and negligible carbohydrates.

BCAAs and leucine

Above we discussed the high content of branched-chain amino acids in whey as one of its important features. Both BCAAs and leucine are available as separate supplements. These supplements can be used to promote muscle growth, with the caveat that since essential amino acids are also necessary for muscle growth, and BCAAs represent only 3 of the 9 essential amino acids, they should be taken with a meal that contains other complete protein, which generally means animal protein – meat, fish, eggs, and dairy. Suggested BCAA dose: 1 to 2 grams, once or twice a day, with meals.

Avoiding muscle loss and infections in illness and aging

When people are hospitalized and/or bedridden, they can lose muscle mass at an alarming rate. In one study, healthy older adults lost one kilogram of muscle mass from the lower extremities alone with 10 days of bed rest; undoubtedly total muscle loss including the upper body was much higher.[15] The muscle loss "was associated with large reductions in strength, aerobic capacity, and amount of physical activity", and is caused by decreased muscle protein synthesis. That massive amount of muscle wasting was in healthy people; in the sick elderly, muscle loss could be much worse, and even more so if they are confined to bed for longer than ten days.

This degree of muscle loss is serious business in the elderly, especially so if they are already ill. It's going to take them a long time to rebuild that much muscle, and in the meantime, the loss may seriously compromise their recovery, and even send them into permanent nursing home residency due to frailty.

Fortunately, protein supplementation can largely prevent muscle loss driven by bedrest and/or illness.

The dismal state of hospital nutrition compounds muscle loss. A study examining the nutritional status of hospitalized patients found:

- 40% of the patients were underweight
- a high incidence of protein-energy malnutrition in these patients
- poor nutritional status adversely affects recovery from illness or injury

- undernourished patients lost even more weight
- this problem is largely unrecognized, and most patients get no nutritional support[16]

Hospitals do not understand protein or the importance of muscle loss, and this seriously impacts the health of their patients.

Besides muscle loss, inadequate nutrition leads to a high rate of infections in the hospitalized elderly, and provision of protein and/or amino acids can cut the infection rate dramatically. In 2011, the CDC reports that there were 721,800 hospital-acquired infections in the U.S., and that 1 in 25 hospital patients acquired an infection during their hospital stay.

Trauma patients who received a formula that included whey protein, along with arginine and omega-3 fats, had a nearly 2/3 lower rate of infections along with better nitrogen balance, meaning that muscle loss was lower.[17] Protein supplementation during illness can make a big difference to the outcome.

In addition to infections and muscle loss, the level of serum albumin is an important indicator, or even cause, of disability and death.[18] Patients with low levels of serum albumin have from two (in men) to four times (in women) the risk of death. Albumin is quantitatively the most important protein in blood serum, and *its level is strongly responsive to the amount of dietary protein.*

Many geriatric patients in long-term care have low levels of albumin; this seems to be just accepted as part of being elderly or in the hospital.[19] Facts suggest otherwise. Low albumin levels in older people, whether they are hospitalized or not, may be due in large part to insufficient dietary protein intake.

Hospital food is abysmal, and dietitians are much more concerned about non-issues like saturated fat and cholesterol, and care much less about ensuring that patients get enough protein. On the other hand, hospital diets are loaded with sugar and other simple carbohydrates; breakfasts at a high-end hospital include items like granola with bananas and skim milk, oatmeal with brown sugar, cinnamon buns, and fruit smoothies; lunch and dinner feature fettuccine, chocolate cake, and bread. Keep in mind that these meals are for patients who are often critically ill and elderly, patients who are much more prone to infection and to loss of muscle mass.

Extra protein can make the difference in recovery from an illness and in the prevention of muscle loss during bedrest.

Glutamine, an unnecessary supplement for muscle

Glutamine is a non-essential amino acid; the body makes glutamine and uses it in many important processes. Normally, the body's glutamine production is adequate, but under stressful conditions, such as intense strength training or critical illness, glutamine production may be unable to meet the body's needs, and thus more glutamine may be beneficial. Glutamine supplementation in critical illness may shorten hospitals stays and cut the rate of infections.[20] Note that the most efficacious method of glutamine delivery to the critically ill is parenteral, straight into the bloodstream, a method not available to athletes. (Well, amateur athletes anyway.)

In athletics, however, glutamine has been a disappointment. Athletes who train heavily become catabolic, that is, their bodies enter a state of breaking down rather than building up. Glutamine levels in their bloodstream decline, and they have increased rates of infections, especially in the upper respiratory tract. Glutamine may be connected to lower immune function and more infections.

Unfortunately, glutamine supplementation doesn't prevent immune changes following heavy training.[21] While bolus doses of 20 grams of glutamine appear to be well-tolerated, they don't seem to support immune function or have an anti-catabolic effect. In resistance trained young men, glutamine doesn't affect muscle mass or strength.[22]

Higher protein consumption, however, does prevent catabolism and declining immune function, and provision of extra protein to overtrained and fatigued elite athletes can return them to health and the ability to train at their previous level.

If you train intensely and nearly daily at any athletic activity, whether strength training, running, or a team sport, and become overtrained and/or fatigued, adding extra protein to the tune of 30 grams a day will give you much better results than glutamine.

Omega-3 fatty acids

Omega-3 fatty acids are the kind found most abundantly in fish and fish oil. Supplementation with omega-3 fatty acids augments muscle protein synthesis in older people in response to amino acids.[23] They also increase this response in younger and middle-aged people, so this doesn't appear to be just an amelioration of an aging condition.[24] The doses used in these studies were high: 4 grams of prescription supplement Lovaza, which provided 3.36 grams of omega-3 daily, and that may not be safe for long-term use.

Nevertheless, an intake of the right amount of omega-3 fatty acids can make a difference to muscle growth. It's not possible at this point to say what the minimum necessary would be; I'll discuss omega-3 fatty acids later in this book.

Creatine

Creatine is a naturally occurring substance that's important in generating energy in muscles. Meat contains a high amount of it, and the body also makes its own, about 1 gram a day. Creatine cycles between a low-energy and high-energy form, and comes into play during intense muscle contraction, such as in heavy exercise.

Lots of misinformation has been spread about the safety of creatine, so let's get that out of the way. In normally used amounts, it's safe. A paper on creatine safety published in the journal *Amino Acids* stated that allegations of adverse effects of creatine are "doubtful", and that liver and kidney function show no changes in healthy people, young or old. The report advises against high-dose creatine (more than 3 to 5 grams daily) in those with kidney disease or health problems that may dispose them to kidney disease.[25] Other than that, anecdotal reports of muscle cramps and stomach upset are about all that can be blamed on creatine, and of course lots of other things can cause these as well.

Since creatine allows muscles to perform at a higher intensity, it may be thought that it would also promote muscle growth, and that thought is correct. In a study on creatine added to a regime of weightlifting, those taking creatine had about double the lean mass gains (that's muscle) as those taking placebo, and strength gains were about 50% greater. Supplementation of creatine in this case was done by the use of a loading dose, at 25 grams a day for the first week, followed by a maintenance dose of 5 grams a day for the next 11 weeks.[26] All the participants were young, healthy men who were already doing resistance training, so this effect of creatine is highly significant.

Creatine improves muscle power and strength in older men too. A group of older men, average age 70, gained more than twice as much muscle when creatine was added to a resistance training program as did those who took a placebo.[27] This study also used a loading dose of creatine at 0.3 grams per kg bodyweight for the first 5 days, and then 0.07 grams per kg each day for the remainder of the 12-week program. That's about 21 grams for an average 70 kg (154 pound) man for the loading dose, and about 5 grams for the maintenance dose. Creatine likely helped these older men overcome some degree of anabolic resistance.

Creatine extends lifespan and improves cognitive function in mice.[28] It increased the expression of genes that control growth and protection of neurons, lowered levels of free radicals, and decreased the accumulation of the aging pigment lipofuscin, which has been called the toxic waste of aging. Creatine therefore has the potential for lifespan extension in humans and the improvement of brain function.

Because of its effect on brain function and muscle growth, some researchers have suggested that creatine could be used in the treatment of certain diseases, especially those connected with aging. Among these are sarcopenia, osteoporosis, Alzheimer's and Parkinson's diseases, and type 2 diabetes.[29]

Given its proven effects, anyone interested in muscle growth should be interested in creatine. It's especially likely to be more effective in those with a poor diet and in vegetarians, since they don't ingest much creatine.

Most of the studies on creatine, as we've seen, used a loading dose for the first 5 to 7 days, but that isn't necessary and may be undesirable; creatine builds up in muscle tissue over time. While a loading dose rapidly increases creatine in muscle over a period of a few days, the same levels can be reached with a maintenance dose of 2 grams a day taken for 28 days.[30] It also takes a few weeks after stopping supplementation for creatine to reach normal, un-supplemented levels. Therefore you don't even need to take creatine daily.

Most of the studies have used a form of creatine called creatine monohydrate, which is the most commonly sold type. Newer and more expensive forms of creatine have come on the scene that promise better results, but there's no evidence for that; creatine monohydrate is as good as any.

Purity may be an important consideration when using creatine supplements. Even small degrees of impurity add up since creatine is consumed in gram amounts, more than most supplements. Look for a product that has 99% or greater purity.

How to use creatine

Most academic studies on creatine used a loading dose followed by maintenance, but since loading doses are not recommended for those with kidney problems or the potential for them, and since a maintenance dose builds up over a couple weeks or so to reach the same body levels as a loading dose, use of maintenance dose only is best. A typical maintenance dose is 2 grams a day. Most supplement manufacturers recommend 5 grams a day, but that appears excessive and my preference is always for the minimal dose that will do the job. Timing of creatine is unimportant, since its concentration in muscles waxes and wanes slowly due to a long half-life. One academic study found that 2 grams sufficed for maintenance, and 3 grams was enough to raise tissue levels starting from scratch.[31] There's also some indication that periodically stopping and restarting supplementation of creatine, cycling it say once a month, allows for a higher muscle level overall.

Suggested use: For muscle growth, 2 grams of creatine daily.

Both NutraBio and Creapure creatine are highly pure products at >99% purity.

Muscle, Strength, and Energy – Key Points

- Strength training and protein are the most important factors in building muscle
- Muscle isn't just for bodybuilders but is important for the health of everyone, and especially older men
- Whey protein contains high amounts of BCAAs that grow muscle and enhance recovery
- Protein supplements can help you reach protein goals and overcome

anabolic resistance
- Mass gainers and ready-made nutritional drinks make poor protein supplements
- BCAAs and leucine as separate supplements can promote muscle growth
- Avoiding muscle loss during illness is crucial
- Omega-3 fatty acids and creatine both promote muscle anabolism

3: Testosterone, Libido, and Potency

The difference between the biology and behavior of men versus women is largely governed by hormones, and the hormone testosterone gives men their distinctly masculine characteristics: greater muscle mass, less body fat, facial hair, male pattern baldness (in some cases). Testosterone also affects behavior, leading to greater self-confidence and higher aggressiveness, and is important to sexual function, including the ability to get and maintain erections and to produce sperm.

In the past, most men didn't need to be concerned about their level of testosterone, and in any case, there was little they could do about it. In the present, men should be very concerned about their testosterone, since many forces are acting to lower it, and lower testosterone leads to a lower quality of life as well as health problems.

Two separate issues impact men's testosterone levels in the present day:

1. Testosterone declines with age
2. Testosterone is declining over time.

It's well-known that as men age, their testosterone declines, but how much of this is due to age and how much is due to ill health or poor body composition (low muscle, high fat) is not known.[1] Some 20% of men over the age of 60 are deemed "hypogonadal", i.e. they have low testosterone, that figure rises to 30% over age 70, and 50% over age 80. On the other hand, "exceptionally healthy men" seem to show no decline in testosterone. So, ill health or, conceivably, age alone, may cause the decline.

Don't think you're out of the woods if you're a young or middle-aged man, though. Testosterone levels have been declining over the years; this is "the secular decline in testosterone", and it's been found both in Europe and the U.S.[2] What this means in practical terms is that a man of any age has, on average, a lower testosterone level than a man of the same age did a few decades ago.

Some researchers have suspected that the rise in obesity and diabetes, medications, or even a decline in smoking rates, have caused this decline, yet even after statistical adjustment for these factors, the decline is still evident. Some have suspected an increase in endocrine disruptors, which are common chemicals found in packaging, cosmetic and household products, and the environment; still others have suspected feminism, a decline in male status, and the "war on men".

Testosterone deficiency is a clinical condition, to be judged by symptoms, not by hard laboratory numbers, since testosterone may have different effects in different men, even at the same absolute level. Symptoms include fatigue, depression, loss of muscle mass, increased fat mass, and loss of libido and erectile function. Low testosterone is also associated with heart disease and all-cause mortality.[3]

The Mayo Clinic defines normal laboratory levels of testosterone as 240-950 ng/dL for a man 19 years old or more. However, as many men have sought testosterone replacement therapy in recent years, laboratories have decreased the lower limit of normal so that fewer men fall outside the normal range, and therefore fewer men are deemed to have low enough testosterone to warrant therapy. In many cases, doctors' hands are tied (by their organization or by insurance companies), so that they can't treat any man whose testosterone falls within the official normal range. So, for example, if you have the symptoms of low testosterone, go to your doctor and get tested with a result of 300 (within the normal range), too bad, you don't officially have low testosterone, so no treatment for you.

There's also been controversy about testosterone replacement therapy (TRT), some studies finding increased rates of heart attacks with it, and others not. This adds to the reluctance of most doctors to prescribe TRT. In this book, however, all the methods of increasing testosterone are done using over-the-counter supplements that increase *endogenous* testosterone, that is, they allow the body to produce more on its own by giving it the right tools for the job.

So, how do you increase testosterone?

Before we get to that, let's look at how you can *decrease* your testosterone. There are a few main ways to decrease it:

1. High fat mass and low muscle mass (i.e. obesity or the skinny fat phenotype)
2. Alcohol
3. Exposure to endocrine disruptors

To understand how they do this, we need to consider the operation of an enzyme called aromatase. This enzyme converts testosterone to two different kinds of estrogen, estradiol and estrone. These two are normally considered female hormones, but they are also necessary and important in men, but men have much lower amounts. If aromatase is more active or abundant, more testosterone is converted to these two forms of estrogen, and the result is a double whammy: less of the male hormone, more of the female. Both obesity and alcohol can increase the production and activity of aromatase.

The solution to the increase in aromatase from alcohol is easy: drink less of it. The solution to obesity isn't as easy though, and that's because low testosterone can cause obesity, and obesity can cause low testosterone, in a feedback loop. If you are obese and have low testosterone, there's no easy way of knowing whether the obesity or low hormones came first. If you attempt weight loss without effect, that might suggest that low testosterone is the cause of obesity.

The extent to which endocrine disruptors lower testosterone isn't known, but they are ubiquitous in packaging (including food packaging) and plastics, and they have the potential to do so.

High doses of exogenous testosterone reliably cause increases in muscle, even without strength training, but even more so with it.[4]

Maintenance of a healthy testosterone level is important for men's sexual health, overall health, and well-being. As we noted, men who are deemed exceptionally healthy may not even experience a decline in testosterone as they age, which shows that good overall health is linked to a healthy male hormonal status. Health status may cause much of the reported decline in men's testosterone levels with age, more so than age itself. As men age, they typically lose muscle and gain fat, and don't exercise as much, and in my view the decline in physical fitness and in body composition affects testosterone more than age.

Besides the supplements listed below, then, the first item on the list to increase or maintain testosterone is to get into good shape. Lose fat, build muscle, do some high-intensity interval training, don't eat sugared junk.

Zinc

We require many minerals for optimal health, but some of these rarely call for supplementation, since we get adequate amounts from food. Calcium, for example, is one of those, as are iron and copper, which we'll cover in a later chapter on supplements to avoid. We often can and do lack other minerals, and these can profoundly affect our health as well as our testosterone production. One of these is the metal zinc, which is important not only to testosterone production, but to healthy aging. (I actually hate that phrase "healthy aging", since the essence of aging is increasing susceptibility to ill health; but put it this way, if you want to stay healthy as you grow older, you'll need some zinc.)

Lack of zinc stunts growth, and while severe zinc deficiency has been found in the U.S., it's usually seen more in undeveloped countries that have a high intake of bread, for example in the Middle East. In the developed world, marginal zinc deficiency is more common, and this is also harder to detect. Meat is one of the best food sources of zinc, but other foods, such as bread as noted above, can hinder its absorption from the gut. Over the past few decades, our health authorities have demonized meat because of its saturated fat content (as it turns out, without any good reason), so meat consumption has dropped and the intake of foods that inhibit zinc absorption have increased. Hence more marginal zinc deficiency.

Vegetarians and the elderly are more likely to have a marginal zinc deficiency, the former because of no meat consumption, the latter because of poor diet. Elderly people also appear to suffer from a decline in zinc transport from the gut, and their general lack of zinc can lead to poor immune function. In a study of elderly urban Americans, zinc intake from food was only about 9 mg a day, whereas the recommended daily allowance is 15 mg.[5] Zinc supplementation improved their immune function.

As we age, the activity of the thymus gland decreases, and the gland itself withers away, a process known as involution. As the thymus plays a major role in cellular immunity via the production of T-cells, the decline in mass of the thymus gland leads to impaired immunity in the elderly, among whom infections are still an important cause of ill health and death. Thymus involution also takes place in animals, and an experiment using mice found that supplementing them with zinc completely restored the activity of the thymus gland.[6] To my knowledge, this effect hasn't been duplicated in humans, though it seems it would be worthwhile to study.

Zinc supplementation could conceivably greatly improve the health of older men and women.[7] Instead, they're subjected to a barrage of drugs (polypharmacy). Naturally, almost no doctors are aware of the importance of zinc.

Zinc can prevent cancer by restoring apoptosis, the cell-suicide program that keeps cells from becoming cancerous. In patients with head and neck cancer, nearly 65% were zinc deficient.[8] Long-term zinc supplementation is associated with a massively lower risk of advanced prostate cancer, 65% lower.[9] The link between marginal zinc deficiency and aging makes sense in the light of the hugely higher risk of cancer in the elderly: people aged 65 or more have at least a 10-fold higher incidence of cancer than those younger; cancer deaths are 15 times higher in that age group.[10]

The human body contains two to three grams of zinc, mostly bound to proteins; as with magnesium, over 300 enzyme systems require zinc for proper function.

Zinc levels in the body are strongly correlated with men's testosterone levels.[11] When young men were put on a zinc-deficient diet, their testosterone levels plummeted by 75%. Ouch. When elderly men who had a marginal zinc deficiency were supplemented with zinc, their testosterone levels nearly doubled. Zinc is hugely important in testosterone production.

The importance of zinc comes with the proviso that if you don't have a marginal zinc deficiency, more zinc won't increase your testosterone, a fact that supplement manufacturers fail to tell you. The supplement known as ZMA, for example, is popular for increasing testosterone. But in healthy young men, it had no effect in raising male hormone levels.[12] Another study using a combination of resistance training and zinc supplementation in healthy young men found no change in hormones, body composition, strength, or endurance.[13]

Nevertheless, older, especially elderly men, are more likely to suffer from a marginal zinc deficiency. It's difficult to test for such a deficiency, since blood levels of zinc don't accurately reflect whole-body stores of it.

Dosage of zinc supplementation can be tricky, since long-term use of a dose higher than the recommended daily allowance can be toxic, manifested by low copper levels. (An established method of treating high copper levels is the use of high-dose zinc.) The tolerable upper intake level of zinc, as set by the U.S. Food and Nutrition Board, is 40 mg a day, while the recommended daily allowance for adult men is 11 mg.

If you have low testosterone levels, zinc could help. Do not exceed the tolerable upper intake level of 40 mg daily, which includes food. The most common form of zinc as a supplement is zinc gluconate, and along with zinc citrate, is superior in absorption to zinc oxide, which in some people is hardly absorbed at all.[14] One way to supplement zinc without going overboard is to take 25 mg a couple times a week. That way you can ensure that you are not marginally deficient, and have all the zinc you need to keep testosterone at optimal levels, without exceeding upper intake limits and risking toxic zinc levels.

How to use zinc

Zinc gluconate is the cheapest and most common form of zinc, and often comes as a 50-mg dose. That exceeds the tolerable upper intake limit, so break or cut the tablet in half, and take one half of a tablet a couple times a week if desired. If you have demonstrated low testosterone, your doctor may prescribe a higher dose.

Magnesium

Unlike zinc, magnesium has little risk of toxicity, but there are probably more people with magnesium deficiency than zinc.

Magnesium is essential.

In the latest study from which data is available, a huge number of Americans, 68% of them, were found not to consume enough magnesium, less than the RDA.[15] Those who consumed less than the RDA for magnesium had a 50% greater chance of having elevated levels of C-reactive protein (CRP), a measure of inflammation, and those who consumed less than half the RDA had a 75% greater chance. Overweight or obesity added to the risks of low magnesium. Inflammation is elevated in disease and aging, and lack of sufficient magnesium could be behind much of it.

Why is magnesium deficiency so widespread? Partly that's due to low consumption of foods that are high in magnesium; these include nuts and shellfish. The high magnesium content of nuts – real nuts, not peanuts – could be one of the main reasons that nut consumption has consistently been associated with better health and longer life. High intake of processed junk food may also be behind widespread magnesium deficiency, since these are low in magnesium, and grains and cereals (including breakfast cereals) impede its absorption.

Hard water also contains a good deal of magnesium, and people are increasingly not drinking it. Numerous studies have found associations between high levels of magnesium in drinking water and lower rates of heart disease, including sudden death.[16] Sudden cardiac death, in which the victim basically just drops dead on the spot, kills hundreds of thousands of people annually, most of them men. Low magnesium is strongly associated with sudden cardiac death, with those in the highest category of magnesium having 40% less risk than those in the lowest.[17] To my mind, that alone is a good enough reason to be taking magnesium.

Low magnesium excretion in the urine, which is a proxy for dietary intake, is associated with increased risk of ischemic heart disease, about 60% higher in the lowest quintile of intake.[18] But no association was found between serum (blood) magnesium and heart risk, and the reason for that is important. The body stores most of its magnesium within the cells and in the bones, about one half in each, with only about 0.3% to be found in the blood serum. That means that blood magnesium levels are a poor indicator of total body magnesium status. Serum magnesium is the most common lab test for this mineral, but if you wanted to get more serious, there's a test for red blood cell magnesium, which has a better correlation with total body magnesium. Most labs will perform a test for RBC magnesium, and it isn't expensive.

More than 300 enzymes in the human body require magnesium as an essential cofactor; these enzymes coordinate and control protein synthesis, muscle and nerve function, energy production, blood sugar, and blood pressure. Metabolic pathways for ATP and mitochondrial energy production crucially require it. Disease states associated with magnesium deficiency include not only heart disease, but hypertension, insulin resistance and diabetes, obesity, anxiety and depression, osteoporosis – and that's not even a complete list.

Take the twin mental health problems of the modern age, anxiety and depression. Both are associated with low magnesium.[19] Animal studies have shown that deficiency leads to anxious, depressive-like behavior, and that giving the animals magnesium alleviates the behavior. In humans, magnesium supplements appear to alleviate depression. Doctors treated elderly women who had low magnesium with 450 mg a day of magnesium, and another group received imipramine, an old-line antidepressant drug. After 12 weeks, both groups saw a decrease in depressive symptoms, with no difference between groups.[20] The researchers concluded that magnesium and imipramine were equally effective in fighting depression. Another study using case histories (but no control group) showed rapid recovery, within 7 days, of major depression using magnesium at 125 to 300 mg with each meal and at bedtime.[21] The effectiveness of magnesium in treating depression requires more clinical research, but given the low toxicity and low price of magnesium, supplementing it seems a worthwhile thing to do in cases of depression.

Oh yeah, what about testosterone?

Magnesium levels in older men are strongly and significantly associated with testosterone levels: the higher the magnesium, the higher the testosterone.[22] (Magnesium is also related to levels of IGF-1, or insulin-like growth factor 1, the growth hormone that's responsible for muscle mass and brain function, among other things.) Magnesium supplementation at 10 mg per kg of body weight (700 mg daily for the average 70-kg man) increases both free and total testosterone in athletes and in sedentary men.[23]

With testosterone in a secular decline, is it possible that lower magnesium levels and widespread magnesium deficiency could be contributing factors?

Magnesium has a huge effect on exercise, as you might expect, since it provides the critical cofactor for so many energy production and enzyme systems. In novice weightlifters, those who took magnesium supplements experienced greater gains in strength than those who did not. The dose used was enough to bring total magnesium intake, including diet, to 8 mg/kg bodyweight, or about 560 mg for a 70-kg man.[24]

Magnesium is a limiting factor in exercise, so to train at your optimum you should make sure you get enough.

However, as with zinc, if you have enough magnesium, more of it will not raise testosterone levels or increase exercise performance, so in that sense, it's not an ergogenic aid. There's a lot of hype out there on supplements and their effects testosterone and exercise, so you need to keep that in mind. On the other hand, with close to 70% of the population not getting enough magnesium, make sure that you're not among them.

Magnesium has a low risk of toxicity. Toxic levels usually only occur in people with poor kidney function, which is uncommon in young, healthy men, more common in old. As with all supplements, and especially for those with some risk of toxicity, consult a doctor before using. (That applies to everything in this book.)

The recommended daily allowance (RDA) of magnesium for a man 19 years old and up is 400 mg.[25]

Magnesium comes in a number of different forms, bonded with different ions or with amino acids or other molecules, for example magnesium citrate, or oxide, chloride, aspartate, and sulfate. These all have varying effects, so the type you get is important.

Epsom salts are magnesium sulfate, and the fact that this compound is used as a laxative tells you a lot about it and about magnesium in general. Magnesium sulfate is poorly absorbed form the gut; it attracts water, hence its laxative function. Milk of magnesia, another laxative, is magnesium hydroxide.

Magnesium can be absorbed through the skin, and some people advocate bathing in Epsom salts to do this; while this can be useful, the main problem with it is that you won't know how much you're getting, whether too little or too much. Magnesium chloride comes in a liquid formulation, to be applied to the skin, but that suffers from the same problem as Epsom salts.

Oral magnesium formulas vary widely in their absorption from the gut, so getting the right kind is critical. Drugstores usually carry magnesium oxide on their supplement shelves, and that form of magnesium is next to worthless. Several studies have found next to zero absorption of magnesium oxide.[26] Magnesium citrate has been consistently found to be the most highly absorbed form of magnesium.

If supplementing with magnesium, get magnesium citrate. It's readily available (online, for example) but your local store may not have it. It usually contains 200 mg magnesium per tablet or capsule. (Also, don't confuse the total weight of the tablet or capsule with the magnesium content.) Powdered magnesium citrate is also on the market, and this works well, as it's cheaper and has little taste.

Magnesium deficiency can cause insomnia, and magnesium has a relaxing effect. Many people report better sleep with magnesium, even a complete cure of insomnia. Even if you don't have poor sleep, taking magnesium at bedtime makes a good option.

One of the surest signs of magnesium deficiency is muscle cramps, especially during sleep. My own muscle cramps completely disappeared when I started taking magnesium at night.

Drinking alcohol and stress can both cause magnesium depletion, so if either of these apply to you, consider taking it.

If you are severely magnesium depleted, it can take a long time, perhaps months, to replete body magnesium stores. The reason is that all of the tissues in the body use it, but don't absorb it at the same rate. It takes time to be distributed and for cells to absorb it. Keep that in mind if you feel that you don't get immediate results.

How to use magnesium

1. Magnesium citrate is the best absorbed.
2. Consider 200 mg magnesium at bedtime.
3. Magnesium has a low risk of toxicity. Supplementing at 400 mg a day appears safe for those with normal kidney function.

Citrulline, erectile dysfunction, male fertility, and exercise

Erectile dysfunction – the inability to get or sustain erections, or to get hard enough erections – increases on average as men get older. It's also associated with insulin resistance and heart disease. Fortunately, there's an over-the-counter supplement that can help, and that's citrulline.

Citrulline is an amino acid that's not used in protein synthesis. The body metabolizes citrulline into arginine; arginine stimulates nitric oxide (NO) and the release of growth hormone; nitric oxide is the factor that lowers blood pressure, keeps blood vessels supple and circulation flowing, and is crucial in erections.

Arginine has been shown effective in raising NO levels and cardiovascular function; NO improves endothelial function, the crucial factor in keeping arteries from becoming stiff and sclerotic, and therefore has uses in hypertension, atherosclerosis, and diabetic vascular disease. So why not just take arginine?

Unfortunately, oral dosing of arginine is very ineffective, because an enzyme in the intestines called arginase breaks it down, and this enzyme increases even more the longer arginine is taken. Citrulline, on the other hand, has no corresponding enzyme, so it's readily absorbed orally, converted in tissues to arginine, and increased NO production results. Paradoxically, taking arginine is not a good way to raise arginine.

Citrulline is also a potent ergogenic aid in exercise; makes sense, since increased NO promotes blood vessel dilation.

In erectile dysfunction, in a study of 24 men, average age 56, with mild erectile dysfunction, took either 1.5 grams of citrulline or placebo daily for one month. It was a cross-over study, so all the men took part in both placebo and citrulline segments in turn. In the treatment arm, 50% of the men reported an improvement in erectile function, compared to 8% of the men in the placebo arm. Frequency of intercourse rose from 1.3 per month at baseline to 2.3 at the end of the treatment phase. The researchers concluded that although it was less effective than drugs such as Viagra, citrulline was well-tolerated and is safe, and should be considered by men who don't wish to take drugs.[27]

Citrulline has a role in sperm quality and male fertility as well. A combination of citrulline, arginine and Pycnogenol®, when given to 50 sub-fertile men for one month, increased sperm volume, motility, vitality, and morphology significantly when compared to placebo. The index of fertility rose to normal values, the activity of nitric oxide synthase increased, and no adverse effects were reported.[28] Which ingredient in this mixture did most of the work is hard to say; Pycnogenol is an extract of French maritime pine bark, and is rich in flavonoids, much like grape seed extract; citrulline on its own may be capable of doing most of the heavy lifting for a task like this.

Citrulline has other benefits too. It can lower blood pressure, increase exercise capacity, and has some potent effects against heart disease. It can even extend lifespan.

Reduced availability of arginine is associated with high blood pressure in both animals and humans; citrulline could therefore be of use in treating hypertension.[29]

Animal studies have shown that citrulline significantly improves exercise performance[30], and in humans who complained of fatigue but who had no evident health problems, citrulline improved muscle metabolism and lowered fatigue.[31] In high-intensity anaerobic exercise – like weightlifting – citrulline improves performance, allowing those who took it to perform more repetitions.[32]

Perhaps best of all, in animals (rats), citrulline decreased the death rate (from 20% to 0% during the course of the experiment), gave them from 14 to 48% more muscle mass (depending on the muscle), and 13% lower fat mass. Besides all that, it prevented lipid oxidation, meaning that one of the primary processes of aging was decreased. Therefore, citrulline looks like an interesting life-extension drug.

Wrapping it up, potential benefits of citrulline include:

1. Lower blood pressure
2. Higher exercise capacity
3. Less fatigue
4. Better erections
5. Improved sperm quantity and quality
6. Better body composition

How to use citrulline

Citrulline comes in powder or capsule form. Doses are not standardized and are not known with any precision. In the study on erectile function, the men took 750 milligrams twice a day. In the study on fatigue, the subjects took 6 grams a day of citrulline malate, which in some formulations amounts to 4 grams of citrulline and 2 grams of malate.

Citrulline has a relatively short half-life of 60 minutes, so it should be taken in divided doses, perhaps twice a day, or shortly before the effect is desired, either before an exercise session or before intercourse.

Citrulline has a good safety profile, but toxicity limits are not really known. As it can cause a decline in blood pressure, anyone who takes blood pressure medications should use caution before using it, i.e. talk to your doctor first.

DHEA

DHEA stands for dehydroepiandrosterone (don't worry, there won't be a quiz). DHEA is an abundant steroid hormone produced by the adrenal cortex and is a precursor molecule to both testosterone and estrogen. Men (and women) have peak levels of DHEA when in their 20s, but those levels dramatically decline with age, such that an 80-year-old may have only 10 to 20% of the levels of his or her youth. Oddly, the function of DHEA isn't at all clear; while aging and DHEA both correlate with increased fat mass, loss of muscle and bone mass, as well as diabetes and heart disease, cause and effect aren't known. The fact that young people have high DHEA, and old people do not, would seem to argue that it's important.

Older men in their 70s who supplemented with DHEA at 50 mg daily had an approximately 50% increase in testosterone.[33] They lost over one kilogram of fat, increased bone mineral density, and gained about half a kilogram of lean mass; these changes may have occurred because of an increase in the growth hormone IGF-1.

Another study using 50 mg of DHEA in older men and women, from 40 to 70 years old, found no rise in testosterone, but of great interest, most of both the men and women reported "a remarkable increase in perceived physical and psychological well-being."[34] However, they had no increase in libido.

Other studies have found similar results, but some have not. Results may depend partly on the age of the participants; younger people have no deficiency of DHEA, so supplementing them with it will do nothing. In older people, DHEA replacement seems to work.

DHEA appears to be relatively safe; a trial of 50 mg DHEA in post-menopausal women, for one year, "did not significantly alter lipid profile, insulin sensitivity or adversely affect the endometrium in postmenopausal women."[35]

DHEA may produce benefits in older men and women, but likely has little to no effect in younger people, i.e. don't expect muscle gains or increased testosterone unless you're over 70.

Boron

Boron is a mineral that is apparently required; "apparently" because not much is known about human requirements. Steady-state excretion in 18 healthy men ranged from 0.35 to 3.5 mg a day, giving some idea of the range of intake required, while supplementation with 10 mg resulted in most of it being recovered in urine.[36]

A couple of studies have found that boron supplementation increased testosterone by about 25% and decreased estradiol by over 30%.[37] However, others found only somewhat increased testosterone, but increased estradiol significantly (see note 36). A study of bodybuilders given boron found that it made no difference in testosterone or lean body mass.[38]

It's likely the case that a boron deficiency decreases testosterone, and correcting that deficiency also corrects testosterone, upward. Several of the studies were done in Iran, the same place where lots of zinc deficiency can be found, and boron helped them. The study on bodybuilders was done in the U.S., and possibly indicates no deficiencies, at least in that group. The jury is still out on whether boron is worth taking.

Aromatase Inhibitors and Testosterone

Aromatase inhibitors can be used to increase testosterone, but before we discuss their use, we need to understand how they work.

Men produce both testosterone and two different types of estrogen, estradiol and estrone. All three hormones are made in the same biochemical pathway, toward the end of which is the enzyme aromatase, which converts testosterone to either of the two forms of estrogen.

The master regulator of testosterone production is a hormone made in the brain called luteinizing hormone, or LH. Both testosterone and the estrogens provide negative feedback on LH in turn. Thus there's a finely controlled mechanism for testosterone production: when there's enough testosterone, LH is dialed back.

The most important feedback inhibitor of LH, however, is estrogen. If the enzyme aromatase, which converts testosterone to estrogen, is too active, then a man has too much estrogen, which feeds back on LH, and testosterone levels decline. High aromatase therefore packs a double whammy, leading to high estrogen and low testosterone.

The main factor leading to high aromatase is excessive fat tissue. It's commonly said that aging increases aromatase, but that's probably due to nothing more than men putting on more fat as they get older.

Certain compounds can inhibit aromatase, lowering estrogen and boosting testosterone. Over 300 natural products have been found to inhibit aromatase.[39] Among the most active products are green tea, cocoa, and coffee.

The polyphenols in red wine also inhibit aromatase.[40] Among these polyphenols are resveratrol and grape seed extract, both available as supplements.[41]

Diindolylmethane, or DIM, found in cruciferous vegetables, is one of the most potent aromatase inhibitors.[42] In high doses, DIM seems to be able to activate aromatase production; therefore DIM should be approached with caution and only a minimal amount taken if desired. Perhaps a better approach would be to eat vegetables that contain it, such as broccoli and cabbage.

Grape seed extract or green tea might prove better approaches to aromatase inhibition, as these compounds are not as potent. Someone who drinks tea and coffee and eats chocolate would also get a fair amount of aromatase inhibition.

Although this is a book on supplements and not drugs, it's worth mentioning for the sake of education that prescription aromatase inhibiting drugs are available, such as anastrozole (Arimidex). Clomiphene (Clomid) is another prescription drug that can raise testosterone, although it works not through aromatase but by blocking estrogen receptors. Most doctors are reluctant to prescribe these drugs to healthy men, though they appear safe enough in low doses. However, some doctors will, so if you have low testosterone with high estrogen, it may be worthwhile to look around for a doctor who will prescribe them. They make for a much cheaper and more hassle-free intervention that testosterone replacement therapy (TRT), since aromatase inhibition requires talking a pill only 2 to 3 times a week, while TRT normally requires injections, is more expensive, and needs more medial monitoring. TRT and aromatase inhibitors are not completely interchangeable interventions, however, so depending on individual need, one may be more suitable than the other.

Vitamin D

We'll have much more to say about vitamin D in this book, but here we'll note its importance to testosterone and men's sexual health in general.

Vitamin D is not so much a vitamin as a steroid hormone. It's made from cholesterol by the action of sunlight on the skin.

Vitamin D is strongly associated with testosterone levels in men. Men who had sufficient vitamin D levels (>30 µg/L) had significantly higher testosterone levels than those with insufficient levels (20 to 20.9) or deficient (<20).[43] As always correlation (or association) doesn't mean causation; perhaps men in ill health and consequent low testosterone didn't get out in the sun as much and thus had less vitamin D in their system. The key point is whether supplementing with vitamin D raises testosterone.

Sure enough, vitamin D deficient men who also had low testosterone saw their testosterone levels increase when supplemented with vitamin D.[44] Total testosterone increased about 30%, and free testosterone about 20%, in men who took 3300 IU vitamin D for one year. Those are solid increases.

Vitamin D receptors are found in the male reproductive tract, and levels of the vitamin are positively associated with sperm motility, making vitamin D an important factor in male fertility. Animal studies found that vitamin D increased fertility. Vitamin D is obviously very important to men's sexual health.

Vitamin D deficiency is widespread, and getting enough sunshine to promote adequate levels of vitamin D can be difficult. In the winter, at higher latitudes, in people with dark skin, sunshine may not be intense enough to synthesize adequate vitamin D. Then there's the fact that many of us are cooped up in offices all day, and are not out hunting or on the farm as in days of old, so we don't get as much sun exposure.

As with zinc and magnesium, if you have enough vitamin D, adding more won't increase testosterone, but many people are vitamin D deficient, so if you need more testosterone, vitamin D could help.

The only way to tell whether your vitamin D is adequate is a blood test; that being said, many men will benefit from supplementation. Vitamin D typically comes in 2,000 IU and 5,000 IU doses; while high vitamin D can be toxic, toxicity is not usually seen except with doses much higher than 10,000 IU daily taken for several months. The Endocrine Society delimits the safe upper intake level as 4,000 IU daily, while the Vitamin D Council, an advocacy group, puts tolerable upper limits at 5,000 IU daily. Dose depends on body weight, initial vitamin D level, whether you get any sun exposure, and other factors. I take 5,000 IU several days a week in the winter, less in summer. (I weigh 160 pounds, and last I tested my vitamin D, it was a satisfactory 60 μg/L.) Vitamin D is extremely important for general health as well, as we'll see.

Oil-based forms of vitamin D are better absorbed from the gut, so get that form. Dry forms of vitamin D may have significantly less absorption.

If you take away nothing else from this book, be aware of the necessity of enough vitamin D. It's that important.

Maca

Maca is a plant from the Andes in South America, and the root has been traditionally used as a medicine by the people who live there. It's related to the cruciferous vegetables such as broccoli.

One of the traditional uses of maca is as an aphrodisiac, a stimulant of sexual desire. Evidence that it works is scanty, but there is some.[45] Maca may relieve sexual dysfunction in men and women who take an SSRI antidepressant. Somewhat more solid evidence, since you can't fake this stuff, is that maca improves semen parameters, including volume, motility, and sperm count.[46] In rats, it reduces prostate size in benign prostatic hyperplasia.[47]

The odd thing about maca is that no one seems to know how it works. It does not raise testosterone. I suspect that, because it's related to cruciferous vegetables, maca may work through a general increase in stress defense enzymes, i.e. through hormesis, so someone who takes other supplements such as berberine or resveratrol may not see much of an effect. But if you suffer from any of these sexual problems, maca may be worth a try. The fact that it improves semen parameters argues for efficacy in that area.

Maca appears to have low toxicity, but exact toxicity doesn't seem to be known. Since it likely works via hormesis, low doses may be all that's necessary.

Testosterone, Libido, and Potency – Key Points

- Ensure that you're not deficient in zinc and magnesium. Supplementing with them is a low-risk strategy providing you stay within upper intake limits.

- Citrulline can improve body composition, and by doing so, increase testosterone. Also lowers blood pressure, increases exercise capacity, lessens fatigue, and in rats, decreases mortality.
- Vitamin D levels are key for testosterone and men's sexual health. Make sure your vitamin D levels are adequate, and if not, get more sun exposure and/or supplement with vitamin D.
- DHEA may raise testosterone in older men who have low DHEA

4: Omega-3 Fatty Acids

Polyunsaturated fats are those in which the carbon bonds in fats are not fully "saturated" with hydrogen. They come in 3 main types, omega-3, omega-6, and omega-9, and the first two are the more important for this discussion. Omega-6 fats are predominantly found in seeds and grains and products made from them or fed with them; vegetable oil contains high amount of omega-6, as do certain animal foods that come from grain-fed animals, of which chicken has the most. Omega-3 fats are also found in some plants; in the animal world, fish has the highest amount of omega-3 fats.

In the course of human evolution, humans ate foods such that they got a ratio of omega-6 to omega-3 fats of perhaps 2:1 or 1:1, and these ratios promote good health and do not promote chronic diseases. In the modern world, due to the presence of vegetable oils and processed food (most of which use vegetable oils in their production), the ratio of omega-6 to -3 fats has shot up to 20 to 25 or even more.[1] This highly lopsided ratio may lead to heart disease, diabetes, obesity, and cancer, as well as effects on brain function.

Omega-6 fats are in general inflammatory, which can account for the association of excess amounts with disease; omega-3 fats are anti-inflammatory.

While the ratio of these polyunsaturated fats is important, so are absolute amounts. It's virtually impossible not to get enough omega-6 fats, so excess amounts of them should be avoided. Large sources of omega-6 fats include vegetable oils, nuts and seeds, and anything made with them, such as mayonnaise and salad dressing and processed foods of all kinds. Flour is made from seeds, the seeds of grain. For better health, these foods should be minimized or avoided altogether.

Omega-3 fats are another story; it may be difficult to get enough in the diet. Since fish – wild, not farmed fish – are the main source of beneficial omega-3 fats, and many people don't eat much fish, the result is a highly skewed ratio of omega-6/3 fats, leading to poor health. Some plant foods such as flax seed contain omega-3 fats of a different type, and these must be converted by the body to the two main omega-3 fats, EPA and DHA; the efficiency of conversion is low, however, so consumption of these foods doesn't guarantee sufficient omega-3 fats.

Heart disease rates differ greatly between different countries, and this may be related to the amount of omega-6 and omega-3 that people consume. In the United States and Europe, the omega-6/3 ratio is about 50:1, and the death rate from cardiovascular disease is 45%; in Japan, where the ratio is 12, cardiovascular death is 12%.[2] There is an inverse relation between fish consumption and coronary heart disease. In Japan alone, those who consumed the most fish, at 180 grams (more than a third of a pound) a day, versus those who consumed the least at 23 grams a day, had about half the risk of coronary heart disease; dietary intake of omega-3 fatty acids – as opposed to just fish consumption – was strongly linked to less heart disease, at a 65% lower rate.

Yet even the lowest level of intake of omega-3 fats in Japan is still about twice the average intake in the U.S.[3]

The effects of omega-3 fatty acids result when cells incorporate them into their membranes. This has led to the idea of the omega-3 index, which measures omega-3 fats in red blood cells as a percentage of total red blood cell fatty acids.[4] An omega-3 index of <4% was found to be undesirable and in a high risk category for coronary heart disease; 4 to 8% was intermediate; and >8% is considered to be in the lowest risk category.

How important is the omega-3 index? The chart below shows 4 quartiles of the omega-3 index and the risk for primary cardiac arrest; the lowest quartile of the index is set at a relative risk of 1.0. (Chart is redrawn from data in reference 4.) The top quartile of omega-3 index had a nearly 90% lower risk of cardiac arrest than the lowest quartile.

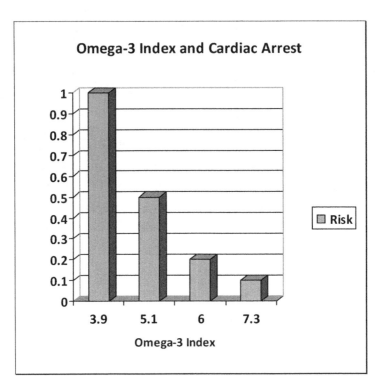

1Omega-3 Index and Relative Risk of Cardiac Arrest. Redrawn from data in Harris, William S. "Omega-3 fatty acids and cardiovascular disease: a case for omega-3 index as a new risk factor." *Pharmacological Research* 55.3 (2007): 217-223.

The omega-3 index is clearly related in a dose-response manner to the risk of sudden cardiac death, so much so, that the inventors of the index calculated that all other risk factors, such as total cholesterol, triglycerides, HDL, and others, pale in comparison.

Omega-3 fatty acids have also been linked to lower rates of cancer.[5] While animal studies and mechanistic (cell culture) studies provide good evidence for their role in the prevention of cancer, human epidemiological studies have been ambiguous, some of them finding lower cancer rates, others finding no effect. But populations with the highest intakes of omega-3 fatty acids, such as in Japan and Greenland, have low incidence rates of prostate and other cancers. The rate of prostate cancer in Japan is only one-tenth that of the U.S.[6]

Total death rates, that is, death from any cause, are lower in people who consume fish regularly, 12% lower in those who consume 60 grams a day, a tiny amount.[7]

Omega-3 fatty acids are anti-inflammatory, and many chronic health conditions involve inflammation, including cardiovascular disease, diabetes, cancer, rheumatoid arthritis, and depression.

People who consume fish have nearly a 20% lower risk of experiencing major depression.[8] Omega-3 fatty acids added to standard therapy in patients with major depression resulted in "highly significant benefits" compared to placebo after only 3 weeks of treatment.[9] Other studies have found similar effects.[10] Lower amounts of omega-3 in red blood cells were found in depressed patients, and the severity of their depression correlated with the level of omega-3.[11]

How to Get More Omega-3 and Improve the Omega-6/3 Ratio

If you find the evidence that omega-3 fatty acids can prevent disease and improve overall health compelling, as I do, then the next step is to increase your intake and your omega-3 index.

As we've discussed, the ratio of omega-6 to omega-3 fats may be just as, or possibly even more important than, the absolute amounts present. Therefore, the first step in improving (decreasing) the ratio of omega-6/3 polyunsaturated fatty acids should be to decrease the amount of omega-6 fats that you consume. Anything made with grains or seeds, and especially concentrated fats from them, contain abundant amounts of omega-6 fats. That indicts primarily vegetable oils, which are better called industrial seed oils.

The most common vegetable oils are canola, soybean, corn, safflower, and peanut oils, although that's not an inclusive list. Most of these oils were all but unknown until recent times, when food companies developed methods of extracting them on a large scale. Their use has skyrocketed in the past century and today amounts to around 70 pounds per capita annually. Vegetable oils arguably account for the very lopsided and dangerous-to-health omega-6/3 ratio in modern times. They are ubiquitous in processed foods, both fast food and prepared grocery-store food.

Until the invention of industrial seed oils, people cooked with lard and butter, and used olive oil as a dressing.

It's no coincidence that the increasing amounts of vegetable oils in our food supply has coincided with rising rates of heart disease and cancer. Unfortunately, health authorities have recommended using these oils for our health, and people have followed that advice. They in fact damage health.

Eliminate them from your diet in order to decrease your omega-6/3 ratio.

Olive oil is not only acceptable but a healthy addition to the diet. Olive oil is *not* an industrial seed oil, but the oil of a fruit that has been known and used since ancient times. For cooking, you can use butter, lard, tallow, or coconut oil.

You'll also need to avoid most processed food. That means things like French fries, tortilla chips, and baked goods like donuts and pastries.

The next step in improving your fatty acid ratio is to eat fish. Fatty fish like salmon is loaded with omega-3 fats, lean fish like tuna less so. Sardines make an excellent choice. If you eat fish two to three times a week, and avoid industrial seed oils, that may be all you need to do.

However, if you're like me, maybe you don't eat much fish. In that case, consider supplementing with fish oil.

You should pay attention to a couple of aspects of supplementing with fish oil to optimize your intake of omega-3 fatty acids: type and dose.

Fish oil capsules should be avoided.

A characteristic of any polyunsaturated fat is easy oxidation, creating byproducts that may harm health, and this applies to fish oil too. Fish-oil capsules sit on shelves at room temperature at the store, and in fact may be subject to much higher temperatures during shipping. Those high temperatures, along with the high surface-to-volume ratio of a capsule, allow oxygen to attack the oil inside its capsule and oxidize it.

Liquid fish oil is my preferred way to supplement fish oil. The oil is sealed inside the bottle, often with an overlay of nitrogen gas to prevent oxidation. After opening the bottle, you should refrigerate it to prevent oxidation. Cod liver oil is the most common type of liquid fish oil and is what I use, though others are fine. Krill oil appears to be more bioavailable – the body is better able to use it – so lower doses can be used than with fish oil. It's more expensive though, so I don't see any great advantage to using it rather than cod liver oil.

Look for a brand that says it's been "molecularly distilled" to remove potential contaminants like mercury and dioxins.

One teaspoon of cod liver oil contains about 1150 milligrams of omega-3 fatty acids, about 500 mg as EPA and 650 mg as DHA; that's about equal to the amount in one can of sardines. By way of comparison, 100 grams (just under a quarter pound) of wild salmon has about 2000 mg of omega-3 fats; only wild salmon counts, as farmed fish contains little.

Next comes the question of dosage. In the case of omega-3 fatty acids, just as with other supplements, more is not always better.

Recall that omega-3 fats are anti-inflammatory. As inflammation is a function of the immune system, excessive omega-3 fats can compromise immune function, and this has been seen in subjects who took fish oil daily; the effect was fully reversible.[12] Of course, this result implies that the same thing would happen if you ate one serving of fatty fish daily, and to my knowledge, that's never been shown. Fish consumption is robustly associated with better health. Men who consumed an average of 35 grams of fish daily had a 42% lower risk of heart disease death than men who consumed no fish at all.[13] It's possible that the lowering of immune function means an improvement in health markers in some situations, and not so in others. Nevertheless, we need to be aware of the possibility.

Eating fish several times a week (averaging to 35 grams daily) greatly decreases the risk of heart attack, and that amount of fish yields approximately 500 mg of omega-3 fatty acids, the amount in about half a teaspoon of fish oil. However, 35 grams of fish daily may not be optimal; they eat much more fish in Japan, where the highest consumers ate 180 grams daily. And Japanese men have much lower risk of heart disease, despite a smoking rate twice as high as in the U.S.

So, a compromise may be necessary in the amount of fish oil with which to supplement, enough to help, not enough to harm. My own compromise is to take a teaspoon of cod liver oil, but not daily, perhaps 3 to 4 times a week. That's the equivalent of eating several servings of fish, or perhaps a half pound of salmon (or 4 cans of sardines) which is enough to greatly decrease my heart disease risk, but not enough to compromise immune function.

Another side effect with very high amounts of fish oil is an increased bleeding tendency; this has been seen for example in Greenland, where fish is a staple, and seems unlikely to affect many people who occasionally eat fish or take fish oil. Nevertheless, if you take any medication to prevent blood clotting, or have any bleeding tendencies, you should consult with your doctor before adding fish oil to your supplement regime.

Omega-3 – Key Points

- The ratio of omega-6 to omega-3 fatty acids is important, as are absolute amounts. We consume far too much omega-6
- Higher levels of omega-3 in cells are associated with much lower heart disease risk

- Omega-3 fatty acids protect against cancer and major depression
- Don't eat anything made with industrial seed (vegetable) oils, such as canola, corn, safflower, soybean, etc.
- If you don't eat much fish, consider taking a fish oil supplement
- Liquid fish oil is better than capsules
- Taking one teaspoon of cod liver oil a few times a week lowers heart disease and other health risks
- Don't overdo it.

5: Weight Loss

Some supplements can help with weight loss when combined with exercise and, especially, diet. If not so combined, it's doubtful that any supplement will help you much. There's no magic weight loss pill, despite what some people claim, and any weight loss from a supplement alone is likely to be minimal.

I'm a big fan of low-carbohydrate diets. Not only do they help most people to lose weight, but they appear to be a uniquely healthful way to eat, through maintaining normal blood sugar and good insulin sensitivity. The amount of carbohydrates in any particular low-carbohydrate diet varies considerably; a diet can't really be called low-carbohydrate unless it has 130 grams daily or fewer. But even given that, *any* restriction of carbohydrates, no matter how small, can be beneficial for health.

Ketogenic diets are those in which carbohydrate consumption is kept very low, usually less than 50 grams, sometimes under 30 grams. These diets result in the production of ketones, which are alternative fuel sources made from fat. While a ketogenic diet is low-carbohydrate, low-carbohydrate diets are not always ketogenic; it depends on just how many grams of carbohydrate one eats.

In contrast, the average American eats nearly half of his or her calories as carbohydrate, or around 300 grams. That's a lot and, in my opinion, is intimately connected to the obesity epidemic.

Regarding exercise, you should give up the idea of "burning" calories by exercising. It doesn't work, since exercise makes you hungry and it's very easy to eat as many or more calories as you "burn". While exercise has many health benefits and everyone should exercise, it unfortunately has a poor record at weight loss when done on its own. Just so you know.

As this is not a diet and exercise book, that's all I have to say for now on those topics. (But see the last chapter.)

When people want to lose weight, what they really mean is that they want to lose fat. For all but the most freakishly large muscle men, excessive muscle is not a problem. Unfortunately, when you lose weight by going on some kind of a diet, muscle loss usually ensues to some degree or other, and that's something to avoid, since muscle loss means worse health. A rule of thumb for weight loss is that *from one quarter to one third of the weight that's lost is muscle*. To lessen or eliminate muscle loss during a weight-loss program, two things work, and ideally you should do both:

1. Strength training – the subject of my book *Muscle Up*.
2. More dietary protein.

Muscles need protein to grow and also need it merely to maintain themselves, since muscle tissue "turns over", that is, it breaks down and rebuilds on a daily basis. Without adequate protein, muscles don't rebuild themselves entirely, and muscle loss ensues. Compounding this problem, on a weight-loss diet, you need more protein than usual to keep from losing muscle.

Protein can also effectively lessen hunger. A good deal of evidence has led to the so-called protein leverage hypothesis of obesity, which holds that organisms, including humans, strongly regulate the amount of protein they consume.[1] If foods are low in protein, an animal will eat more of the food to satisfy its protein requirement; hence, low-protein foods can lead to obesity. The converse of the protein leverage hypothesis is that foods high in protein can lead to eating less and to weight loss.[2] High protein foods also lead to higher thermogenesis after a meal, meaning that the metabolic rate increases and more calories are burned.

The greater satiety (less hunger) seen with a high-protein diet leads to decreased energy intake of several hundred calories daily.[3] That's a recipe for weight loss in itself.

Using whey protein as a supplement can increase your protein intake without providing too many calories, since whey is almost pure protein, and it can help to preserve muscle.

In a study of weight loss, subjects were placed on a diet that provided 500 fewer calories a day than they normally ate. One group consumed 10 grams of whey protein twice a day, once before breakfast, and once before dinner. Both groups, whey and non-whey, lost similar amounts of weight, but the whey group lost significantly more fat and less than half the amount of muscle. Of the weight loss in the non-whey group, over *half* was muscle, while the whey group lost only about 20% of their weight as muscle.[4] (NB: Throw in some weightlifting or other strength training, and you could keep muscle loss to zero.)

In obese older (average age 63) adults, the addition of 21 grams of whey protein at 10 times a week, to a low-calorie diet, resulted in similar weight loss to those who didn't use whey, but the whey group *gained* muscle while the non-whey group lost muscle.[5]

The quality of protein intake, as well as the number of times a threshold for protein is reached daily, correlates strongly with the amount of abdominal fat.[6] Abdominal fat in turn is strongly associated with metabolic abnormalities; it's the worst type of fat for health. High-quality protein contains a high fraction of essential amino acids. Adding whey or casein protein as a supplement could help you lose abdominal fat.

How much protein do you need while eating a low-calorie diet in order to preserve muscle mass? One study found that those who ate more than 1.2 grams of protein per kilogram of body weight were significantly more likely to keep their muscle than those who ate less; for fat-free (lean mass), that worked out to 1.9 g/kg daily.[7] So, for example, if you weighed 200 pounds and were 25% body fat, your fat-free mass is 150 pounds, and you should eat about 130 grams of protein a day to preserve muscle while on a reducing diet. Probably the best way to get enough protein without adding a lot of calories is with whey protein.

To lose weight and preserve muscle, you can either add whey to meals, or use whey as a meal substitute for one meal a day. A typical dose of whey is 20 grams, which could be used as a once-daily meal replacement; if adding to meals, you can use 10 grams.

Please keep in mind that the type of protein under discussion here is whey protein, and other types, such as casein, may work well. *Don't use meal replacement shakes or drinks, such as Ensure, Boost, Slim-Fast, or other, similar drinks.* Not only are they not terribly high in protein, the factor that most keeps hunger at bay, but they're a witches' brew of sugar, vegetable oil, and chemicals. Among the first few ingredients in Boost, for example, are sugar, corn syrup, and vegetable oil, foods that not only have deleterious effects on metabolism, but which are precisely the foods you should avoid if you're trying to lose weight. It's a shame that those meal replacement products are considered food and complete sources of nutrition, especially so since older and ill people tend to use them the most.

For the best type of whey to use for weight loss, see the section on whey in the chapter on muscle.

MCT Oil

MCT stands for medium-chain triglycerides, which are a unique form of fat; coconut oil, which has many health benefits, contains a high amount of MCTs. About 60% of the fats in coconut oil are MCTs.[8]

Triglycerides are fats, and when ingested, they are either stored as fat or burned as fuel. Triglyceride molecules have long chains of carbon atoms, so triglycerides can be designated as short, medium, or long chain. Medium-chain triglycerides, MCTs, are much more readily burned than short or long chain fats. The liver can also use them to make ketones, which can then fuel the brain and other tissues.

MCTs raise the metabolic rate much more than long-chain triglycerides. Oxygen consumption, a measure of the metabolic rate, was 12% higher after ingestion of MCTs, compared to 4% higher after LCTs. In addition, MCTs resulted in a 25-fold increase in beta hydroxybutyrate, which is the most important ketone body, but no effect of LCTs.

MCT oil as part of a weight-loss diet led to greater weight loss than a similar diet that included olive oil. The dieters that included 18 to 24 grams (around 1 to 2 tablespoons) of MCT oil lost nearly 4% of their body weight in 16 weeks, as opposed to the olive oil group, which lost less than 2%.[9] Animal studies have also shown that MCT oil decreases the amount of body fat mass.

MCT oil works either by its thermic effect – more calories burned than stored – or by increasing satiety, or both. In some ways, MCT oil can mimic the effects of a ketogenic diet by increasing the level of ketone bodies in the bloodstream. However, on its own, the effect of MCT oil is likely to be small; in other words, don't expect great weight-loss results if your only effort is taking it.

MCT oil, as a product, is a concentrated source of MCTs, 100% compared to the 60% of coconut oil.

MCT oil and Bulletproof Coffee

Bulletproof Coffee, which tech executive Dave Asprey has made popular in recent years, contains both MCT oil and grass-fed butter. Asprey claims that his coffee "provides fast energy with no crash". Is there anything about claims that have been made for Bulletproof Coffee?

Bulletproof Coffee (BPC) has both pluses and minuses. On the plus side, coffee alone does provide a jolt of energy. When MCT oil and butter are added, the addition may make for less hunger. Because of this, many have started to use BPC in place of breakfast, and if used this way, it could help weight loss, even though it has a couple hundred calories or more. Coffee aids the practice of intermittent fasting, so when that's the case, BPC can work well, I believe. On the other hand, coffee, either black or with a tiny bit of cream, also aids intermittent fasting with only a fraction of the calories. On the other, other hand, BPC is likely to be a lot healthier than a bowl of sugar-laden cereal for breakfast.

Asprey claims that the MCT oil in BPC, by increasing levels of blood ketones, aids the brain, specifically by giving you better focus and energy. That may be, as ketones can improve mitochondrial function both in the brain and the rest of the body. If you always eat a clean diet and are lean, BPC might give you some edge. Otherwise, the results may be underwhelming, because other factors in your diet (sugar for instance, or refined carbs) may negate benefits on brain function from MCT oil.

As for grass-fed butter in BPC, it is indeed healthy, but there's no reason you have to put it in coffee. Just use it in place of regular butter. (Also, throw out your industrial seed oils, like corn and safflower oils. They cause cancer and heart disease; virtually all processed food is made with them too.)

I doubt Asprey's claims about mycotoxins. While mycotoxins are real, whether the amount in coffee is enough to care about is another question, and I very much doubt the claim that special coffee with no mycotoxins helps you think more clearly.

As for MCT oil alone, there's some evidence that they can help with weight loss. Use sparingly, perhaps one tablespoon at a time. Some people report digestive upset, so be aware of that. Coconut oil, which contains a high amount of MCTs, is great for cooking, as it can be heated to high temperatures without burning. Merely using coconut oil in place of your usual cooking fat or oil may give you enough MCTs to make a difference in weight loss.

Fat-Burning Supplements

Fat-burning supplements raise the metabolic rate and thus burn more energy, the idea being that you will lose fat by burning it.

Fat burners are a bad idea. For one thing, diet is by far the most important factor in fat loss, and taking a pill or other supplement to burn fat is unlikely to help much.

For another thing, there have been a number of reports of toxicity in people who use them.[10] While these appear to be uncommon, the risk hardly seems worth it. In people with heart problems, fat burners can increase heart rate and blood pressure enough to precipitate real danger.

Your best shot at fat loss is a sound diet, cutting out all sugar and flour and vegetable oil. Exercise, while it won't "burn" calories enough for weight loss, improves insulin sensitivity and builds muscle, which are important for fat loss. High levels of insulin keep fat inside fat cells; when insulin declines, fat can leave these cells for use as a fuel source. Adding protein as suggested above can ratchet back hunger.

Weight Loss – Key Points

- The most important factor in weight loss is food
- When losing weight, do not lose muscle, as that results in worse health. It's muscle you may never get back

- Adding protein to your diet can help you retain muscle
- High-quality protein intake means less abdominal fat
- MCT oil may help fat loss
- Bulletproof Coffee? Maybe
- Don't take fat-burning supplements.

6: Longer Life

The supplements discussed in this book can improve health, or increase the odds for better health. In a very real sense, that means that supplements can slow aging. Why is that?

Aging by definition means an increasing propensity to ill health and disease. As the body ages, damage to cells and tissues accumulates, and they become less able to maintain normal physiological functions and to defend the body from a stress. The aging body has a tendency to break down. If we can stop the body from breaking down with time or when faced with a stress, such as an infection or a high amount of physical activity, then we've effectively slowed or even reversed aging.

Scientists have been avidly studying the causes and effects of aging for decades, even hundreds of years when looked at broadly. While much work remains to be done, we appear to be on the verge of real breakthroughs in the science of aging, and with them, the ability to slow or reverse the aging process.

To understand how some substances, whether drugs or supplements, can slow aging, we need to know what causes it. While scientists have not fully elucidated these causes, we do now have some major clues about how aging happens.

One of the biggest clues lies in the phenomenon of calorie restriction (CR). Scientists discovered as long ago as the 1930s that restricting the amount of food that a lab animal eats results in an extension of its lifespan. That's a counterintuitive result for anyone that thinks about aging, since it might logically seem that giving an animal *more* food would allow it to repair itself better and to withstand the stresses of life. Instead, CR of from 10 to 40% less food causes an animal to turn on stress response and repair genes that result in longer life.

Scientists have written and published thousands of papers attempting to explain how CR works. Among their theories are

- CR results in less pro-aging fat tissue
- CR deactivates mTOR, a physiological engine of both growth and aging
- CR increases stress defenses
- CR changes the microbiome, the totality of microorganisms that live in and on the body
- CR lowers the metabolic rate

There are many other theories on how CR works. But the key idea here is that CR is a sort of archetype of anti-aging, since it's the most robust and reliable method to extend the lifespans of lab animals. Once we understand how CR changes the physiology and biochemistry of animals, that opens the field to chemical compounds that have the same effects. Any substance that acts like CR would be a *calorie-restriction mimetic*, in effect a drug that slowed aging.

CR causes a stress response, which leads to the wider idea of *hormesis*.

Hormesis is the process through which low doses of a toxin or stressor cause an organism (plant or animal) to become stronger, while higher doses are toxic and cause weakness, ill health, or death. Perhaps the most obvious example of hormesis is exercise: by pushing the body to a level of intense physical activity greater than what it's used to, the body becomes stronger and better able to withstand the same amount of activity the next time it occurs. Muscles grow bigger, the heart pumps more strongly, and oxygen is better delivered to the tissues where it's needed.

Besides CR and exercise, other examples of substances or processes that cause hormesis are radiation, fasting, and a number of natural compounds that we'll be looking at.

Scientists have discovered several drugs that can slow aging, the two most important being rapamycin, an immunosuppressant drug used in organ transplant patients, and metformin, the most widely prescribed anti-diabetic drug in the world. While rapamycin shows great promise in slowing aging, it has major side effects that preclude it from being used, at least for now; current work on this drug shows that "pulse dosing", for example once a week, may give most of its benefits with fewer of the unwanted side effects, but much more work needs to be done before humans can use it. There's currently a large trial of rapamycin in pet dogs.

Metformin also shows great promise. Metformin lowers blood glucose (sugar) and insulin, and people who take it have lower rates of cancer. It causes weight (fat) loss, and it extends lifespan in rats. Metformin comes from a plant whose medicinal uses have been known for hundreds of years, and it's cheap and not patented. As we'll see, there's an over-the-counter, non-toxic, and inexpensive supplement, also known for hundreds of years, that may work as well as or even better than metformin.

Unlike drugs, the supplements discussed in this chapter have a low risk of toxicity, they're relatively inexpensive, act through many of the same mechanisms as anti-aging drugs, and are available without prescription.

Resveratrol

Resveratrol, a substance found in grape skins and in red wine, has been the subject of a great deal of controversy and hype over the past couple of decades, after it was found to prevent cancer in cell cultures and in animals.[1] Scientists also discovered that it could extend the lifespans of two common lab "animals", the tiny worm *C. elegans*, and the fruit fly. Unfortunately, it failed to extend lifespans of mammals, such as rats and mice, dashing hopes that resveratrol would be the next big thing in aging and health.

Resveratrol does, however, have many interesting health benefits; for example, mice who were fed a high-calorie diet lived longer when also given resveratrol, and their physiology shifted to be more like those fed regular food.[2] Obese humans given resveratrol at 150 mg a day for 30 days had a decreased metabolic rate, indicating that the compound functions as a calorie-restriction mimetic. Resveratrol activated AMPK, the important cellular energy-sensing program, it increased the activity of mitochondria, the powerhouses of the cell, and somewhat improved markers of insulin resistance.[3]

In animals (rats), resveratrol enhanced exercise performance and augmented the benefits of exercise alone. According to the authors of the study, "Resveratrol, an antioxidant found in red wine, has beneficial effects on cardiac and skeletal muscle function, similar to the effects of endurance exercise training."[4] That means that resveratrol is an exercise mimetic.

Also in rats, resveratrol doubled sperm counts and increased levels of testosterone.[5] It may be worth taking for that reason alone, although the effect hasn't been shown in humans.

Resveratrol retards the aging of neuromuscular junctions, which metformin failed to do.[6] Resveratrol in this case acted as a calorie restriction mimetic.

On balance, I believe resveratrol is well worth taking as a supplement, and I do take it. Resveratrol appears to have low toxicity at doses that have been used in humans, for example at 150 mg a day in the study on obese people, but doses are not known with any certainty. Bioavailability appears low, that is, resveratrol is rapidly metabolized and excreted, leading some observers to state that achieving physiologically significant levels might be difficult; however, resveratrol metabolites may be active as well, and it's not even established that high levels in the circulation are necessary for beneficial effects. One way in which resveratrol works is through transformation of the gut microbiome, the mix of bacteria that reside in our intestines, and for this effect, gut absorption isn't even necessary. Some researchers believe this could be the most important effect of resveratrol.[7]

Commercial resveratrol supplements typically contain up to 500 mg per capsule, but that's usually a 50/50 mixture of *cis* and *trans* resveratrol, and only the *trans* form is active. Since resveratrol acts via hormesis, that much may not be necessary.

What about resveratrol in red wine? A bottle of red wine contains perhaps 10 mg of resveratrol (amount varies), so getting, say, 250 mg of resveratrol would require drinking 25 bottles of wine, a difficult, undesirable, and possibly fatal task. Don't do that. Resveratrol probably isn't entirely responsible for the health effects of red wine, which is loaded with other polyphenols from grapes; these polyphenols, along with alcohol, likely are responsible for a great deal of the benefits.

Will resveratrol give you longer life? That's unknown, and any life-extending effect may be minimal. But it does have health benefits, and it seems a low-risk way to get some insurance. As mentioned, though it appears safe, doses are unknown, so exercise caution. A low dose of 20 mg exerts beneficial effects, and 100 mg perhaps more.[8]

Vitamin D

We discussed vitamin D in the section of testosterone and men's sexual health, but vitamin D is also very important for better overall health and longer life. So, let's discuss it a bit more.

Vitamin D is produced by the action of sunlight on the skin, so it's not really a vitamin, since there's no dietary requirement; it's actually a hormone. It can be taken as a supplement, and it's present in some foods; fish and fish oil are the biggest dietary sources. It helps promote strong bones and prevent rickets, which for a long time was thought to be its only action. Vitamin D promotes the absorption of calcium and phosphorus from food, and these elements are important in bone and overall health.

Rickets, the softening of bone, is only the most extreme manifestation of vitamin D deficiency. While less than the optimal amount of vitamin D won't necessarily cause rickets, it will affect the immune system, muscle, and the brain, as well as cardiovascular health and cancer. Vitamin D deficiency is usually defined as a blood level of <20 ng/ml, insufficiency as <30, and sufficiency as >30. (Note that sometimes the units of nmol/L are used to measure vitamin D, and this can be confusing. To convert nmol/l to ng/ml, divide by 2.5.) The only way to know for certain whether you are deficient or sufficient in vitamin D is through a blood test. Most labs can perform one.

Vitamin D levels are negatively associated with mortality from cardiovascular disease.[9] One problem with associations like this one is that obesity correlates negatively with vitamin D, and outdoor activity correlates positively, and both of these are also associated with heart disease. However, most of the evidence shows that vitamin D levels are still (negatively) associated with heart disease after adjustment for CVD risk factors. Randomized controlled trials of vitamin D supplementation have been inconclusive, however.

Women with breast cancer are more likely to have lower vitamin D levels than those without. A study of vitamin D supplementation in post-menopausal women who took vitamin D and calcium found a massively lower rate of cancer of any kind, about 60% less.[10] (Curiously, calcium alone also lowered cancer rates, a result that doesn't agree with studies showing that calcium supplementation is associated with higher death rates.) The women took 1100 IU of vitamin D daily, for 4 years.

An analysis of vitamin D trials found that vitamin D concentrations greater than 40 ng/ml (100 nmol/L) were associated with more than 65% lower risk of cancer.[11] (The analysis was confined to women only.)

Higher rates of cancer seen among African-Americans, in overweight and obese people, and in regions where there's less solar radiation points to an association with vitamin D.[12]

Large epidemiological studies have shown that low vitamin D is associated with significantly higher death rates.[13] Some studies of vitamin D supplementation have shown no benefit, but many of the earlier studies were marred by low doses of the vitamin, such as 400 IU, a dose now known to be grossly inadequate to substantially raise D levels in the body.

Low vitamin D levels are associated with depression.[14] Depressed people who supplemented with vitamin D and were low in it to start with had a significant improvement in their condition.[15]

Vitamin D deficiency has been described as epidemic, one reason being that many of us don't get enough sunshine; in the past, outdoor work such as farming was much more common, whereas now most of spend much of the day working indoors. Obesity is associated with low vitamin D, and this may be because the vitamin is sequestered in fat tissue and becomes unavailable to the rest of the body; with more obesity around, this could lead to greater incidence of deficiency. While supplementing vitamin D is effective at raising levels, many people are unaware of it. People with dark skin who live in northern latitudes may not be able to make enough vitamin D when exposed to the weaker sunshine there.

Get some sun

Ultraviolet radiation from the sun is the major source of vitamin D for most people, since the only significant dietary source is fatty fish (see ref. 9). Exposure to the sun for enough time, and with sufficient intensity, to produce a slight pinkness to the skin (which is called a minimal erythemal dose) produces about the equivalent of 20,000 IU vitamin D, i.e. a fairly large dose. The amount of time spent in the sun to do this varies considerably with latitude and season of the year. At a latitude above 37 degrees north, which in the United States runs roughly between San Francisco, California, and Richmond, Virginia, sunshine is not strong enough to produce vitamin D in the skin other than in the summer. Furthermore, to get that 20,000 IU of vitamin D from the sun, minimal clothing and a mid-day time period are required. With all of this, it can be seen that many people in the U.S. and elsewhere are at risk of deficiency.

Sunshine may be the best way to get enough vitamin D, because exposure to solar radiation has other benefits besides. The action of sunshine on the skin raises the level of nitric oxide (NO), which is a very important blood vessel dilator that's highly correlated with good arterial health. It lowers blood pressure and protects against cardiovascular disease. Safe sun exposure is important, since excess sun on the skin can lead to skin cancer; but the benefits of sun exposure far outweigh the risks, since far more people die of heart disease than skin cancer, of which the non-melanoma type is rarely fatal. Skin cancer is a marker for sun exposure, and people diagnosed with skin cancer have a nearly 50% reduced risk of death from any cause – sun exposure is that powerful.[16] In fact, "*avoidance of sun exposure is a risk factor for death of a similar magnitude as smoking.*[My emphasis.] Compared to the highest sun exposure group, life expectancy of avoiders of sun exposure was reduced by 0.6–2.1 years."[17]

So, while vitamin D is important and supplementing it can be of great benefit, it probably can't entirely substitute for getting regular, safe sun exposure. Over the past few decades, mainstream health authorities have bombarded us with warnings to stay out of the sun, which, while it prevented many cases of skin cancer, may have actually increased the death rate. Safe sun exposure is important; avoid sunburns, and if you plan to be out in the sun a long time, by all means use sunscreen.

A recent review of vitamin D made the following points (ref. 7):

- Vitamin D deficiency is a global health problem
- Vitamin D is important in immunity, cardiovascular disease, and cancer
- Lowest mortality rates are seen at a level of 30 to 45 ng/ml (75-100 nmol/L)
- It's reasonable to maintain vitamin D levels at 30 to 60 ng/ml

The Endocrine Society, an association of doctors and scientists in endocrinology, suggests that adults may need 1500 to 2000 IU of vitamin D daily to maintain a blood level above 30 ng/ml. They also suggest a tolerable upper limit of vitamin D for "maintenance" of 4,000 IU daily for adults, "not to be exceeded without medical supervision", while acknowledging that higher doses may be needed to correct deficiency.[18]

However, and this is a big however, a couple of scientists calculated that the Institute of Medicine made a huge mistake when it estimated the recommended dietary allowance for vitamin D.[19] In their new calculation, the scientists calculated that for 97.5% of individuals to achieve vitamin D blood levels of 20 ng/ml (50 nmol/L), as much as 8900 IU of vitamin D per day might be needed. The authors state, "As this dose is far beyond the range of studied doses, caution is warranted when interpreting this estimate. Regardless, the very high estimate illustrates that the dose is well in excess of the current RDA of 600 IU per day and the tolerable upper intake of 4000 IU per day." While that dose (8900 IU) is high, and most people probably wouldn't need that much, it does show the serious underestimation of vitamin D requirements.

Vitamin D supplementation can be tricky, since there are so many variables involved, such as your latitude, the season, your initial vitamin D level, your skin color, and whether you get much outdoor time. The only way to find out if you have enough vitamin D is through a blood test.

In the summer, assuming you get outdoors relatively often and get sun exposure, supplementation may not be necessary; the body stores vitamin D to last for several months, so if you get enough in summer, you may, again depending on a lot of variables, have enough to get you through the winter. My own current practice is to take 5,000 IU perhaps 3 to 4 days a week in the winter, and less in the summer. Of course, what works for me won't work for everyone, as I'm light-skinned and live in a sunny part of the country. When I took 5,000 IU daily (in winter), my blood test showed 70 ng/ml, which may be just on the edge of too high, so I cut back my supplementation. Getting to very high levels of vitamin D, over 70 ng/ml, may have some deleterious effects, but data is limited.

As noted elsewhere in this book, oil-based forms of vitamin D supplements are absorbed better than dry forms.

Vitamin D Key Points

- Vitamin D is more like a hormone than a vitamin
- Vitamin D is associated with less cancer, heart disease, and mortality
- Sunlight, which produces vitamin D in the skin, is also important for other reasons, so you should get some
- Vitamin D blood levels depend on many factors, such as body weight, latitude, season, and skin color
- Vitamin D RDA may have been seriously underestimated.

Green and Black Tea

Green tea, which is commonly drunk in China and Japan, is associated with lower rates of cancer, about 30% lower in those who drank the highest amounts of green tea compared to the lowest. Deaths from cardiovascular disease were about 25% lower in the highest consumption group versus the lowest.[20] This is of course epidemiological evidence, meaning that it can't show whether green tea actually prevented disease, or that there's some other connection such as that healthier people drank more green tea.

Laboratory and other evidence, however, provides some good reasons to think that green tea is the real deal when it comes to disease prevention.

Green tea contains molecules called catechins, and the most abundant and potent for health purposes is epigallocatechin gallate (EGCG for short, no quiz this time either). EGCG inhibits cancer cells in cell culture (i.e. in a test tube).[21] It prevents tobacco-induced cancer in mice.[22] As the literature on green tea and health is abundant, I'll cite just a couple more.

In one study, doctors gave green tea extract to men with a condition known as high-grade prostate intraepithelial neoplasia. Thirty percent of men with this condition can be expected to be diagnosed with prostate cancer within one year of diagnosis of the first condition. The men in the study were divided into a treatment group, and a control group, the latter getting a placebo capsule. The treatment group took 3 green tea capsules of 200 mg each daily, for a total of 600 mg a day of green tea extract. The capsules were about 52% EGCG, and total catechins about 75%. After one year, only one man in the group treated with green tea extract developed cancer, for a cancer incidence rate of about 3%, whereas among the placebo-treated men, 9 cancers were diagnosed, for a cancer incidence rate of 30%.[23] If the results of this study held true, that could mean that green tea extract may reduce the incidence of prostate cancer in men with high-grade prostate intraepithelial neoplasia by 90%. That result is nothing short of remarkable.

Another study looked at the effects of green tea extract in colorectal adenoma. Similar to the study above on prostate cancer, the subjects had a condition that predisposed them to cancer, namely colorectal adenoma, a benign tumor or polyp. The patients had their adenomas removed, and were then placed on 1.5 grams of green tea extract daily. The control group got no supplements. After one year, the patients were examined for the recurrence of polyps, which was 15% in the treatment group, and 31% in the control group, for a risk reduction of more than 50%.[24] The study's authors stated, "GTE [green tea extract] is an effective supplement for the chemoprevention of metachronous colorectal adenomas."

Green tea extract can improve exercise performance and fat loss. Young men who took 570 mg of GTE for 4 weeks had a 25% increase in fat oxidation (burning for energy), a 1.6% decrease in body fat, and an 11% exercise performance improvement.[25]

EGCG has extended lifespan by more than 10% in rats.[26] Oxidative stress and damage in kidney and liver were lower with EGCG, as was expression of genes that control inflammation.

How does green tea work? As with other interventions, its mechanism of action isn't known with certainty, although it has many biochemical effects. Green tea chelates ("key-lates") iron, meaning that it binds to iron inside the body and removes it.[27] Since cancer is associated with higher iron, that's one way it could prevent cancer.

Green tea catechins also have neuroprotective effects. They promote the increase of stress defense enzymes through Nrf2, a key regulator of these enzymes. Green tea catechins also cross the blood-brain barrier, and have been suggested for prevention and treatment of Alzheimer's and Parkinson's diseases.[28]

However, there's a caveat: green tea extract in high doses could be toxic.

Recent reports claim that green tea extract has caused liver toxicity in some people. While liver toxicity may be uncommon or rare, the severity of this illness means that it should be avoided at all costs. How much can cause damage?

That isn't known with certainty, although a mouse study that caused liver damage used a dose of pure EGCG (1500mg/kg) not likely to be used by humans.[29] Nevertheless, there have been some dozens of cases of human toxicity, so I believe you should just drink green tea and avoid green tea extract.

Many of the studies on the health benefits of green tea found those benefits in people drinking 5 cups daily or more daily. Green tea varies greatly in its catechin content. Japanese matcha tea has the highest catechin content of any green tea, at least three times higher than any other green tea, and 137 times higher than from an ordinary brand of Chinese green tea.[30]

Black tea can also benefit health. Black tea is made from the same plant as green tea, but it's processed differently; black tea leaves are fermented, green tea leaves non-fermented. As a result of fermentation, the catechins in tea leaves become theaflavins, which can inhibit cancer, and may even be more powerful in that regard than green tea catechins.[31] Theaflavins chelate iron and other metals, likely accounting for a great deal of their health benefits.[32] Drinking tea with a meal therefore decreases iron absorption from food, which for most adult men is a good thing.

Consumption of black tea reverses endothelial dysfunction in patients with coronary artery disease.[33] Endothelial cells make up the thin layer on the inside of the arteries, and lack of flexibility in them and inability to respond to stimuli is a sign of stiff arteries leading to coronary disease.

Drinking 3 or more cups of black tea daily is associated with large reductions in coronary heart disease, reductions as much as 70%.[34] Another study found that one cup of black tea daily was associated with 44% lower risk of heart attack.[35] Good Lord, sounds like black tea is the cure for heart disease.

Most of the research on green tea consumption has taken place in the Far East, mainly China and Japan, where more people drink green tea. Black tea is probably just as health-promoting as green, but because it's less exotic, and because most Americans don't drink it, black tea has been ignored, relatively speaking. Both black and green tea can protect against or prevent hypertension and atherosclerosis by improving vascular function.[36] A recent study in Singapore found that daily tea drinking was associated with far less risk of cognitive decline, as much as 80% less in high-risk (APOE e4) carriers, and any kind of tea, black, green, or oolong, was protective.[37]

Some studies have found that milk added to black tea may inhibit absorption of polyphenols, which are thought to account for tea's health benefits. Others have not found any diminishing of tea's iron-chelating ability with added milk. It may be a good idea to drink tea without milk; cream would likely not have the same effect, since there's no protein in it, and that's the constituent that binds polyphenols.

So, go ahead, drink black or green tea, and you'll likely get the same health benefits from either one.

Coffee has its own health benefits, and whether coffee or tea is better is not known, but you could always drink both.

Berberine

Traditional Chinese medicine has used the compound berberine for as long as a couple thousand years, using it to treat infections and diarrhea. Berberine has potent effects against a range of bacteria, protozoa, and fungi. But its benefits against the diseases of civilization have only begun to be discovered in recent years.

Berberine has multiple effects on many biochemical systems, but perhaps the most important is that it activates AMPK, the cellular energy sensor that regulates metabolism from the top down. (Other activators of AMPK include exercise and calorie restriction, making berberine both an exercise and calorie-restriction mimetic.) AMPK shifts metabolism away from growth and toward a state of repair.

Berberine's most important effect may be in lowering blood sugar (glucose), and in this regard, it's been shown to be as powerful as the top-prescribed diabetes drug metformin. In one study, 36 people with type 2 diabetes were assigned to either berberine or metformin, each at 500 milligrams, three times daily. Berberine lowered blood sugar and HgbA1c (a measure of long-term blood sugar levels) as well as metformin. In 48 people with poorly controlled type 2 diabetes, berberine decreased fasting insulin by 28% and insulin resistance by 44%.[38]

If you're not actually diabetic, why should this matter? Higher blood sugar is associated with worse health, even in non-diabetics. In studies in animals, berberine downregulated the expression of genes that promote lipogenesis (the making of fat and storage in fat cells) and increased the expression of genes that regulate energy expenditure.[39] Metabolism was thus shifted from sugar-burning to fat-burning, a healthy metabolic state.

That leads to another benefit of berberine, weight (fat) loss. By improving insulin sensitivity, berberine promotes fat loss, in one study, from a BMI of 31.5 to 27.4. i.e. from obese to non-obese merely from taking berberine and doing nothing else.[40] Whether it would do anything for those already in decent shape isn't known.

Berberine is anti-inflammatory and may prevent cancer; it inhibits the growth of numerous types of cancer cells *in vitro*.[41] It has extended lifespan in one laboratory animal, the fruit fly. It has antidepressant effects.[42]

Berberine has a multitude of effects, but in preventing aging, its stimulation of AMPK and the consequent increase in autophagy may play the predominant role. Autophagy, the cellular self-cleansing process, declines strongly with age, and returning it to normal, youthful levels can slow or reverse aging. As the mechanism of berberine appears to be nearly identical to that of metformin, and it has virtually the same effects as that drug, and metformin extends lifespan in mammals (not just worms), berberine qualifies as a promoter of life-extension.

Berberine may be one of the most potent anti-aging agents that you can buy over-the-counter.

Berberine "is generally considered to be a non-toxic alkaloid at doses used in clinical situations (200–1000 mg two or three times daily)."[43] Berberine capsules generally come in 500 mg doses; powder is also available, but it's intensely bitter, so most people would probably want to use a capsule. (It's about as tasty as chewing an aspirin tablet.) For those who do not have blood sugar problems, taking it once a day may suffice to get benefits. Since berberine works via hormesis, the best bet is to take it sporadically and with minimal dosing.

If you have blood sugar problems or take any medications that influence blood sugar, you should consult a doctor before using berberine.

In short, berberine may be a first-class anti-aging supplement due to its actions on AMPK and autophagy, and its ability to lower blood sugar and promote fat loss.

Curcumin

Curcumin is derived from the Indian spice turmeric, which is typically about 8% curcumin. Unless you eat a lot of curry, a curcumin supplement supplies a more biologically meaningful dose.

Curcumin, like berberine and green tea, modulates numerous biochemical pathways and has anti-inflammatory and neuroprotective effects. It prevents cancer in lab animals and has undergone Phase II clinical trials in humans with pancreatic cancer, where it was well-tolerated.[44]

One of the most significant effects of curcumin, in my estimation, is that it chelates (binds and removes) iron.[45] Since excess iron causes all manner of problems, the ability of curcumin to remove iron is likely related to many of its benefits.

Cell, animal and epidemiological studies indicate that curcumin could be useful in the prevention, and possibly the treatment of:

- Cancer
- Alzheimer's disease
- Parkinson's disease
- Type 2 diabetes
- Rheumatoid arthritis
- Ulcerative colitis
- Major depression

Curcumin is a potent anti-tumor agent and affects multiple molecular targets in cancer. It has activity against virtually every type of cancer cell against which it's been tested.[46] Cancer prevention may be one of curcumin's most important features. Taken with any regularity, curcumin may snuff out nascent cancer cells and since cancer is the number two killer in the U.S., that makes curcumin a powerful life-extender.

In an animal model of dementia (in rats), curcumin decreased oxidative stress and restored memory deficits.[47] Curcumin decreases amyloid plaques in the brains of mice; these plaques are strongly associated with Alzheimer's disease.[48] A recent review on polyphenols and Alzheimer's disease said that "Three compounds are highlighted in this review - Curcumin, Resveratrol, and Epigallocatechin-3-gallate. These compounds have huge potential for AD treatment, especially due to their low frequency of adverse events."[49]

Curcumin is a potential neuroprotective agent against Parkinson's disease. It crosses the blood-brain barrier to exert anti-inflammatory effects.[50] It improves obesity-associated inflammation and diabetes in animals.[51]

In a clinical pilot study, i.e. using humans, 500 mg a day of curcumin significantly treated rheumatoid arthritis, and in fact was better than a standard arthritis medication.[52] Curcumin treatment in this trial was found to be safe and unrelated to any adverse events; the study "provides the first evidence for the safety and superiority of curcumin treatment in patients with active RA [rheumatoid arthritis]."

Curcumin given to patients with ulcerative colitis in remission significantly improved relapse rates.[53] The dose used was 1 gram twice a day.

Curcumin has potential in the treatment of major depression.[54]

Curcumin may treat non-alcoholic fatty liver disease, which is caused by eating sugar, vegetable oils, and lots of refined carbohydrates, has become epidemic, and is closely associated with diabetes and obesity. Rats given a diet designed to give them fatty liver and also treated with curcumin displayed little of the pathological changes in their liver compared to those without curcumin.[55]

Curcumin has low absorption from the gut, and is metabolized relatively rapidly. To fix the metabolism problem, curcumin supplements are often formulated with piperine, a substance from black pepper that decreases the metabolism of curcumin. (Piperine has anti-inflammatory action on its own.) To increase absorption of curcumin, taking it with a meal is best, especially if that meal is high in fat.

The effects of curcumin overlap to an extent with some of the other supplements discussed here. For example, it chelates iron as do IP6 and green tea, and it decreases inflammation like berberine. That leads to the question whether you should take curcumin if you already take, or plan to take, some of the others. Unfortunately, that can't be answered with certainty. Certain health conditions may respond better to curcumin than to others. But the clinical use of curcumin is in its infancy; while it holds a lot of promise and shows efficacy in preventing and treating many conditions, doctors prefer to prescribe drugs. Pharmaceutical companies are uninterested in clinical trials, since curcumin is cheap and can't be patented, hence it won't generate large profits for them.

Curcumin appears safe. A number of clinical trials (that is, using people and not animals) found no evidence of toxicity in people taking up to 8 grams daily for a short period of time, although most of the trials used amounts of from 1 to 2.5 grams daily.[56]

Curcumin typically comes in doses of 500 mg, standardized to 95% curcuminoids (curcumin plus related compounds with biological activity). Be aware of an all-too-common curcumin scam, the selling of the spice turmeric as curcumin. A cursory look online reveals a number of companies that do this, labeling their products as "turmeric curcumin". If it is labeled like that, pass on it. Look for the label to say merely "curcumin", along with "standardized to 95% curcuminoids" or similar wording. If the ingredients are a "curcuminoid blend" whose first ingredient is turmeric root extract, or just turmeric, then it's a scam. You might get some curcumin in it, but it won't be enough, and in any case, you'll pay much more than you need to.

Sidebar:
Coffee, Tea, Red Wine, and Chocolate

The supplements we've discussed here – resveratrol, berberine, and curcumin – are all examples of polyphenols, a class of chemicals found in plants, or phytochemicals. Phytochemicals are, at least in part, what give fruits and vegetables their health effects. They act to upregulate cellular stress defense mechanisms, making cells stronger and better able to withstand injury.

While fruits and vegetables contain beneficial phytochemicals, they are much more abundantly found in four common food and drink items: coffee, tea, red wine, and chocolate. Not surprising, since these are all concentrated plant products.

The consumption of all of these has been associated with lower death rates. In addition to some of the supplements discussed, for better health and longer life, you can freely add any of these items to your diet, with certain provisos. Some people are more sensitive to the caffeine in coffee, tea, and chocolate, and red wine of course contains alcohol, and limits to its consumption should be respected. Chocolate usually contains a good deal of added sugar, so be careful on that score; dark chocolate is the only type shown to have health benefits.

Most people find these food and drink items highly enjoyable, so this is one exception to the general rule that comfort makes you soft and unhealthy. These foods and drinks make you healthier and hardier.

IP6

IP6, or inositol hexaphosphate, is a natural phytochemical derived from rice bran and found in grains and vegetables as well. Also referred to as phytic acid or phytate, it's sometimes considered an "anti-nutrient", meaning that it inhibits the absorption of other nutritional elements. It turns out that those anti-nutrient and other properties make it anti-cancer and neuroprotective. IP6 is cheap and safe.

IP6 has been known for some time to be an anti-cancer agent.[57] IP6 decreases cellular proliferation and differentiation of malignant cells causing them to revert to a normal cell phenotype.

In cell culture, IP6 significantly inhibits the growth of pancreatic cancer.[58] "Our findings [stated the researchers] suggest that IP6 has the potential to become an effective adjunct for pancreatic cancer treatment."

IP6 has been shown to inhibit the growth of colon, breast, prostate, liver, and skin cancer cells.

IP6 also has been proposed to treat Parkinson's disease.[59] In Parkinson's disease, dopamine neurons progressively decay and die, and this appears to be closely related to the content of free iron in those parts of the brain. IP6 chelates iron in a cell-culture model of Parkinson's.

It's been suggested that IP6 may also be able to treat Alzheimer's disease.[60]

One concern about the use of IP6 for Parkinson's or Alzheimer's is that it's ability to cross the blood-brain barrier is unknown, and that would be necessary for it to exert favorable effects on the brain.

Dopamine neurons in all human beings decay and die at a rate that sets an upper limit to human life at about 115 years. The difference with people who get Parkinson's disease is merely that the rate of decay of dopamine neurons is faster: when only 30% of dopamine neurons are left, overt Parkinson's disease becomes apparent, and when only 10% remain, death ensues. For those who don't suffer from Parkinson's, the theoretical point of only 10% of the dopamine neurons remaining comes at age 115.

It follows that IP6, by preventing or perhaps even reversing Parkinson's disease through iron chelation, could extend human lifespan. Indeed, iron restriction extends lifespan in *C. elegans* and in mice. Iron supplementation decreases lifespan in *C. elegans* by promoting protein insolubility, leading to a general sort of gunk of proteins that are needed for life.

As with many other supplements, one reason IP6 is not better known is because it is so cheap and cannot be patented, so drug companies can't make any money from it; therefore they don't fund research into it.

The major mechanism of action of IP6 appears to be that it chelates iron: it attaches to free iron atoms and then both are eliminated from the body. Cancer cells require large amounts of iron to grow and reproduce, and when iron is taken away from them they can no longer do so. This may help explain the Warburg effect, in which cancer cells preferentially burn glucose anaerobically; this might be due to mitochondrial damage from large amounts of free iron.

A recent study found that in mice who were deliberately loaded with high iron, IP6 alleviated oxidative stress and injury to the liver by chelating iron. Ferritin (iron) decreased, and genes for inflammatory cytokines, the chemical messengers which ultimately result in damage, were down-regulated.[61]

IP6 prevents calcification and therefore may prevent kidney stones.[62] Might it prevent abnormal calcification of arteries? That's not known, as far as I'm aware, but it seems an intriguing possibility, in which case IP6 might prevent heart disease.

IP6 is well-tolerated and has showed no toxicity in animal studies. Since IP6 binds iron, as well as calcium and other metals, there remains a possibility that it could lead to mineral deficiencies, but long-term intake of IP6 in pure form or in food hasn't caused them.[63] The U.S. FDA lists IP6 as GRAS, for Generally Recognized As Safe, meaning it's considered non-toxic and can be added to food without any special testing.

Doses are not known with any degree of certainty. The serving size of one of the more popular IP6 products, IP6 Gold, is 3.2 grams of IP6, just to give a ballpark figure. IP6 also comes in bulk, and most people will find this perfectly acceptable, since it has little taste at all.

One-quarter teaspoon is about 500 mg of IP6, and this could be taken first thing on an empty stomach, perhaps first thing in the morning. Taking it on an empty stomach means that the IP6 will not merely chelate minerals in one's food, but will be absorbed into the body where it can chelate iron already there.

As mentioned above, one concern about IP6 is whether it can cross the blood-brain barrier, a relatively impermeable border crossing that allows only select agents across in order to protect the brain. Whether it can do this or not does not prevent IP6 from chelating iron elsewhere in the body and performing its other anti-cancer functions.

Other polyphenols that act as iron chelators do cross the blood-brain barrier, notably those contained in green tea. Unlike with some other supplements, IP6 has unique properties that overlap with other supplements only minimally; therefore, I take it.

Key points

- IP6 has strong anti-cancer properties
- IP6 protects neurons from cell death
- It chelates iron, probably its main mechanism of action
- It may be able to prevent or treat Parkinson's and Alzheimer's diseases

- IP6 is cheap and safe

Lithium

Most people know lithium as the "drug" given to bipolar patients. In reality it is not a drug but a mineral, and in bipolar disorder it's given in high doses: the target dose is on the order of 900 to 1,800 mg a day.

However, lithium is a required nutrient, and evidence suggests a recommended daily allowance of 1 mg a day for a 70-kg adult.[64] As you can see, that's a far lower amount than the dose given in bipolar disorder.

Low levels of lithium in drinking water have been associated with violence, suicide, and homicide.[65] Depending on location, drinking water varies greatly in the amount of lithium it contains, which is how researchers were able to find the relation between lithium and suicide.

Lithium increases lifespan too. Mortality rates in humans are inversely associated with lithium concentrations in tap water; furthermore, the lower mortality rate remained after adjusting for suicide, showing that lithium provides some other health benefit not strictly related to mental health. Since this association does not show causality, the same study tested low-level lithium, at about the same concentration found in the tap water, on the worm *C. elegans*. It extended their lifespan.[66] Lithium appears to be a bona fide life-extension substance.

Lithium may extend lifespan by promoting autophagy, the cellular self-cleaning process that rids cells of junk and is crucial to lifespan extension. It does this by an mTOR-independent mechanism, meaning that it does not depend on fasting. Likely through increasing autophagy, lithium has been found to delay progression of amyotrophic lateral sclerosis.[67]

As stated above, about 1 mg a day is a suggested RDA for lithium. Dose for bipolar patients are hundreds or thousands of times higher, but there's considerable risk of toxicity at those doses, while there appears to be little for low doses. A commonly available formulation, lithium orotate, provides 5 mg lithium. The half-life of lithium, the amount of time it takes for a 50% drop in levels in the body, is about 24 hours. Based on both half-life and common doses, my practice is to take one 5-mg tablet every few days, as insurance that I'm getting enough lithium. Alternatively, the tablet could be cut in half and taken more often.

Aspirin

Aspirin is not usually considered a supplement, but since it's over-the-counter and derived from a plant, and something everyone concerned about his health should be aware of, I'm going to discuss it here. It's important.

It's often said that if aspirin were invented today, it would be considered one of the most important drugs ever made, and also said that if it were invented today, the FDA would never approve it due to its side effects. There's some truth to both of these statements.

For a few decades, many doctors have advised taking low-dose ("baby", or from 75 to 81 mg) aspirin for people at risk of heart disease, and as a result, millions of people have been taking it. (For comparison, a regular-size aspirin tablet contains 325 mg.) However, a couple of facts get in the way of recommending universal aspirin use.

One is that aspirin causes bleeding. The same action that makes aspirin effective against heart attacks and strokes, namely its ability to block the action of blood platelets and therefore to prevent blood from clotting quickly, also increases the tendency to bleed. The major sites of bleeding are the gastrointestinal tract and the brain, and bleeding in either of these places can be serious or even fatal.

The second fact, or at least putative fact, that has put a brake on aspirin use is that it appears less effective, according to some studies, in primary prevention, that is, in people who have not previously had a heart attack. It works best in secondary prevention, which is prevention of another heart attack in people who have already had one.

Nevertheless, the U.S. Preventive Services Task Force currently recommends that men, age 45 to 79 years, be encouraged to use aspirin by their doctors "when the potential benefit of a reduction in myocardial infarctions outweighs the potential harm of an increase in gastrointestinal hemorrhage."[68]

What this means in practice is that if a doctor has determined that if a man has a significant risk of heart attack that is greater than his risk of harm from bleeding, then he should be encouraged to take aspirin.

The back-and-forth on aspirin has been going on for years, at first encouraged, then discouraged, now encouraged with reservations.

Then a strange thing happened. It was discovered that aspirin prevents cancer.

As a result of millions of people taking aspirin for many years, due to the first, encouraging recommendations, plus a lot of people just taking it on their own (for both heart protection and for pain or inflammation), researchers were able to study their health over time, and they found out that those taking aspirin got less cancer. A lot less.

The decrease in cancer risk with aspirin turned out to be large. Early studies were epidemiological, that is, they showed an association with aspirin use and less cancer.[69] That left open the possibility that some other factors could explain the association, such as people with cancer avoiding aspirin, or health-conscious people taking it. But randomized trials of aspirin use to prevent cardiovascular disease had also been done, so researchers took a look to see how much cancer the subjects of these trials got.[70]

In eight randomized trials, aspirin users had a risk of cancer 21% less than those who did not take aspirin. After five years or more of aspirin use, cancer risk was 34% less. In some particular types of cancer, risk reduction was even greater; for instance, risk of gastrointestinal cancer in those who took aspirin more than five years was 54% less. Lower rates of many types of cancer were seen, such as esophageal, pancreatic, colorectal, stomach, lung, prostate, bladder, and kidney cancer. Aspirin also reduced the risk of metastasis, the spreading of cancer from its origin to other sites within the body.

Earlier recommendations on aspirin use had considered only two factors, cardiovascular risk and bleeding risk. Now there was a third factor that needed to be considered: less cancer risk. That changes the equation.

Peter Rothwell, M.D., the physician who has led many of the studies on aspirin and cancer, said, "In terms of prevention, anyone with a family history [of cancer] would be sensible to take aspirin."[71]

If you don't have a family history of cancer, it might still be sensible to take aspirin. A group of researchers have plugged cancer risk prevention into the equation, and created a website into which one can enter one's age, sex, values for cardiovascular risk, cancer risk, bleeding risk, and preferences for how strongly you would like to avoid any particular health problem, and get a result for whether you should take aspirin or not. The site is at http://www.benefit-harm-balance.com/.

Using this site, for men ages 45 to 54, the advice skews heavily against taking aspirin. For this group of men, the risks generally outweigh the benefits, unless the risk of heart disease and the desire to avoid cancer are relatively high. In older groups, over the age of 55, the advice skews much more favorably toward taking aspirin, such that most men would be advised to take it.

Rothwell himself, along with colleagues, estimated the benefits and harms of taking aspirin in the general population.[72] They wrote, "Prophylactic aspirin use for a minimum of 5 years at doses between 75 and 325 mg/day appears to have favourable benefit–harm profile; longer use is likely to have greater benefits. Further research is needed to determine the optimum dose and duration of use, to identify individuals at increased risk of bleeding, and to test effectiveness of *Helicobacter pylori* screening–eradication before starting aspirin prophylaxis."

The biggest reductions in cancer were in colorectal cancer which, depending on the study, was decreased by as much as 52% in those who took aspirin at least 5 years. Esophageal cancer was decreased by as much as 58% with 5 years or more of aspirin use. Another report by a different group found that in men who took aspirin for 5 years or longer, prostate cancer incidence was decreased by 57%.[73]

Recently, researchers found that even short-term use of aspirin could prevent cancer, and a reduction in the incidence of metastasis could be the reason for this.[74]

Aspirin doesn't just prevent cancer, it could even treat it.[75] Aspirin, at doses that appear to be physiologically attainable (i.e. non-toxic), causes oxidative stress in cancer cells, killing them. Those are test-tube experiments, though, and clinical studies have not been done.

Bleeding is the most important adverse side effect of aspirin. Bleeding into the brain, or hemorrhagic stroke, is the most serious bleeding event and is potentially fatal. Estimates suggest a relative increase in this type of event of about 35%, from a baseline rate of 0.03% per year. So, with aspirin, the absolute risk of an intracranial bleed is about 0.04% per year.

Gastrointestinal (GI) bleeding can be severe and also fatal, is more common than an intracranial bleed, but usually is less serious. Aspirin increases the risk of GI bleeding from between 30 and 70%, from a baseline rate of 0.07% per year; with aspirin, absolute risk of a GI bleed rises to about 0.09% to 0.12% a year. Gastrointestinal complications increase greatly after the age of 70, but rates and fatalities are low in those below age 70. People with stomach ulcers, previous bleeding episodes or tendencies to bleeding should NOT take aspirin. Risk factors for bleeding include increasing age, male sex, diabetes, hypertension, obesity, smoking, alcohol consumption, and infection with *Helicobacter pylori*, the cause of stomach ulcers. Rothwell and colleagues write that "restricting prophylactic use [of aspirin] to age <70 years in average-risk individuals may be prudent at this stage. However, since the cancer risk also increases steeply with age, use at older ages may be beneficial if the carry-over benefit of aspirin is limited." ("Carry-over benefit" refers to the fact that aspirin appears to protect from cancer long after people stop taking it.) They also write, "Caution is necessary in prophylactic use in those with high alcohol consumption."

Their final summation:

"In summary, analysis of benefits and harms in the general population in the developed world suggests a net benefit for a minimum 5 years of aspirin prophylaxis starting between ages 50 and 65, for both men and women, with larger benefits for 10 years of use. Continuing aspirin use for a longer duration also appears to be beneficial; however, there is uncertainty about the age at which it should be stopped."[76]

Based on current guidelines, a recent study concluded that only about 40% of people who should take aspirin are in fact doing so.[77] (We don't know how many are taking it that shouldn't be, and that certainly happens.)

What's the verdict on aspirin? That depends on individual circumstances, and given some of the resources here, as well as consultation with your doctor, you can arrive at some reasonable conclusions. Aspirin is most likely to benefit men over the age of 50, and unless other circumstances intervene, it's unlikely to be a net benefit to those under 50.

Aspirin could be one of the more potent life-extension drugs available. It extends the lifespan of mice, who do not get heart attacks but do have high rates of cancer.[78] A research group recently screened a selection of plant extracts that delayed chronological aging in yeast, announcing, "One of these extracts is the most potent longevity-extending pharmacological intervention yet described."[79] The extract was from willow bark, the parent source of aspirin, and it was >25% salicin, the anti-inflammatory compound found there, chemically related to aspirin, and which becomes salicylate when metabolized, the same metabolite of aspirin. It may act as a calorie-restriction mimetic, through activation of AMPK.

Aspirin acts in at least two main ways. Chemically, aspirin is acetylsalicylic acid (hence it's sometimes referred to as ASA), and when ingested, it's rapidly deacetylated to form salicylate. The acetyl group attaches to platelets, deactivating them; this is how aspirin exerts its effect against heart attack. The remaining salicylate relieves pain and extends lifespan.

Low-dose aspirin is a dose of 81 mg, and doses used in the observational studies that I've cited range from 75 mg daily and up to much higher doses. Doses higher than 75 mg do not appear to confer greater health benefits, but they do appear to increase risks, mainly from bleeding.

Aspirin can cause injury to the lining of the stomach, which leads to stomach ulcers. Enteric-coated aspirin, which does not dissolve in the stomach but does so in the small intestine, does not injure the stomach lining. Physical contact of the aspirin tablet with the stomach lining appears necessary for to effect injury.[80] Note that enteric-coated aspirin does *not* decrease the risk of bleeding, which is a separate problem.

Until something better comes along, dirt-cheap aspirin may give as good a shot at a longer, healthier life as any other drug.

Aspirin Summary

- Aspirin may prevent both primary and secondary heart attacks

- Aspirin prevents cancer; in some studies and in some cancers, up to 75% (for esophageal cancer)
- In some animals, aspirin extends lifespan
- Risk of bleeding must be balanced against benefits
- Men under 50 are unlikely to benefit
- Men between 50 and 70 are more likely to benefit
- Men over 70 are likely to have higher risk of adverse effects like bleeding, but they also have higher risk of heart attack and cancer, so doctors are undecided whether this group should take aspirin
- Alcohol use, previous ulcers, and previous bleeding increase risks of aspirin
- Consult with your doctor before taking aspirin on a regular basis

Vitamin K

Vitamin K is a very overlooked micronutrient that can have a large effect on your health, preventing heart disease and cancer. While all vitamins are important, in contrast to most others, people are more likely to consume inadequate amounts of vitamin K.

Vitamin K comes in two basic forms, phylloquinone or vitamin K1, which is found in plants, and menaquinone or vitamin K2, found in animal foods.

In the Netherlands, a study found large differences in heart disease mortality, all-cause mortality, and aortic calcification among subsets of people grouped by vitamin K2 intake.[81]

The relative risk of death from coronary artery disease in the highest tertile (third) of vitamin K2 intake was 0.42; that is, those with an intake of vitamin K2 in the highest third, compared to those in the lowest third, had nearly a 60% reduction in risk of death from heart disease.

Risk of all-cause mortality (death from any cause) was 0.74, or ~25% less, and the risk of aortic calcification was only about half that of the lowest intake group.

Another study found that each 10 μg/day intake of vitamin K2 was associated with ~10% lower risk of coronary artery disease. (Average intake was about 29 μg/day.) The highest quartile of vitamin K2 intake in another study had about a 20% lower risk of coronary artery calcification, in line with the other study's 25% lower rate of aortic calcification.[82]

Worthy of note, none of these studies found that phylloquinones, the vitamin K from plants, had any effect; it was all vitamin K2.

One reason that this is noteworthy is that it seems to rule out the healthy user effect seen in so many studies. The healthy user effect occurs when people who are already healthy enthusiastically follow health recommendations and their subsequent health is misattributed to the recommendation. For example, many studies have found health benefits for low-fat eating, but the people most likely to eat that way are those who are smart, conscientious, and likely to have kept abreast of health recommendations over the past few decades. They're healthier, but not because of their diets. In contrast, those who consumed lots of meat have been more likely to smoke, be overweight, and not exercise.

So, healthy users will have been more likely to eat lots of plant foods, high in vitamin K1, but these were shown to have no effect on mortality. The unhealthy users would have been likely to eat more vitamin K2, and this did show an effect.

Other studies have found lower cancer rates with vitamin K2 consumption.[83] This was a "trend", i.e. not considered significant, at a 28% lower rate of cancer mortality. Cancer risk reduction was more pronounced in men than in women, with a significant inverse association with prostate and lung cancer.

The inverse association between vitamin K2 consumption and lower rates of heart disease makes sense, since one of the functions of vitamin K2 is in calcium metabolism. Calcification of the arteries is a cause of coronary heart disease. Essentially, vitamin K2 gets calcium into the right places, bones instead of arteries. Because of its effect on calcification, K2 can improve teeth too, preventing or even fixing cavities.

How do you get more vitamin K2? One of the studies cited above says that dietary intake of vitamin K2 is "highly determined by the consumption of cheese." K2 is also found in butter and eggs, much more so if these come from grass-fed animals. But this also depends on the season of the year, where the animals are fed and what exactly they eat. Grass-fed butter, for example Kerrygold from Ireland, contains a fair amount of vitamin K2.

To be on the safe side, I take a vitamin K2 supplement, because it's important. For an adult man, adequate intake of K2 is 120 μg a day. Many supplements come in approximately 100 μg doses. Note that one brand, Carlson, comes in a 5-mg size, which is far higher than the daily requirement. I use this brand, but open the capsules and pour out about a fifth of it into my coffee on most days, one capsule lasting me a week.

Vitamin K Summary

- Vitamin K signals for calcium to go to the right place, namely bone
- Lack of vitamin K means calcium can go where it causes harm, namely arteries
- Vitamin K prevents cancer and heart disease
- Grass-fed dairy such as butter and cheese contains a fair amount of vitamin K
- To be sure you get enough vitamin K, a supplement may be worthwhile

Glucosamine

Glucosamine is a supplement commonly used for osteoarthritis and joint pain, although its efficacy in treating these conditions is not firmly established, with the most recent studies finding no benefit. Large numbers of older people take it, an estimated 7.4% of Americans aged 57 to 85. Despite the negative results in clinical trials, lab tests indicate that glucosamine could be anti-inflammatory and thus prevent diseases such as cancer, cardiovascular disease, and chronic obstructive pulmonary disease (COPD, commonly found in cigarette smokers).

To determine whether glucosamine could extend lifespan, researchers looked at data from 77,510 people, aged

50 to 76, who had participated in a study about supplement use, including use of glucosamine.[84]

On follow-up several years later, the use of glucosamine was associated with 18% lower death rate than non-users. When specific causes of death were examined, current use of glucosamine was associated with a 13% lower death rate from cancer, and a 33% reduction in death from all causes. The study found only an association, however, and causation isn't shown.

However, a lab study on aging mice found that glucosamine extended their lifespan.[85] Glucosamine lowered their blood sugar, activated AMPK, and increased the number of mitochondria, leading the scientists to state that glucosamine "extends life span in evolutionary distinct species by mimicking a low-carbohydrate diet."

Glucosamine also activates autophagy, the cellular self-cleansing process, and this could be an important means for its life-extension and anti-inflammatory effects.[86]

How much glucosamine is needed for the lifespan-enhancing effect? Unfortunately, that's unknown. In the study of glucosamine users, the only distinction made was among never users, former users, and current users, and the other studies were of course done on animals. One could speculate that the usual daily dose of glucosamine users was enough to improve their health, although whether more or less would do the job better is not known.

That glucosamine appears to mimic effects of a low-carbohydrate diet has led me to skip the glucosamine supplement, since I already eat in this way and glucosamine would probably be superfluous. It would not affect the biomarkers already affected by my diet more than the diet alone. That's my thinking anyway; since so little is known at this point about glucosamine, amounts required, how it works, and so on, all that we can do is speculate.

Glucosamine Summary

- Glucosamine extends lifespan in animals, and is associated with longer lifespan in humans
- Glucosamine may prevent heart disease, cancer, and COPD
- It extends lifespan in animals by mimicking a low-carbohydrate diet
- Doses are not known with any certainty

Glycine

Glycine is a non-essential amino acid, meaning that we can make it ourselves and therefore it's not an absolute dietary requirement. However, some scientists have argued that we don't or can't make sufficient glycine for optimal health and that getting higher dietary amounts can result in better health.[87] Glycine may indeed be a healthy substance to get more of.

One of the hallmarks of aging is dysfunction in mitochondria, the powerhouses of the cell. Mitochondria have their own DNA, and the mitochondrial theory of aging posits that increased mutations in mitochondrial DNA cause this dysfunction. A neat piece of scientific research found that the respiratory defects in mitochondria are due not to mutations in mitochondrial DNA, but to epigenetic regulation, in other words, due to changes in gene expression.

The Japanese scientists who performed the study found that reversing the epigenetic changes caused the mitochondria in cells from very old people, aged 80 to 97, to become basically like brand new mitochondria, with the functional capability of mitochondria from fetal cells. That's a very good thing and would go a long way toward making someone look and feel younger, and with the better health of youth too.

The scientists found two genes that control mitochondrial respiration, and it happens that these two also control glycine production in mitochondria. When glycine was added to culture media containing cells from the 97-year-old, the mitochondria in these cells became like new.

This study suggests a number of things. One is that aging may be programmed. Mitochondrial dysfunction with aging appears not to be a matter of accumulating mutations that the organism has no control over, but rather a controlled difference in gene expression, controlled by the organism itself. In other words, aging is not accumulation of random damage, but a programmed function.

Aging is a completely natural process, and living "according to nature" won't fight aging; you must outwit nature to increase maximum lifespan.

Two, it suggests that glycine supplementation can fight aging, and indeed, in the experiment, it did, albeit in cell culture, not *in vivo*. It's too early to say what the proper dose of glycine might be, but we can speculate that it would be enough to bring glycine levels up to those seen in young people. (Or even to levels seen in infants.)

Curiously, we already know that in rats, glycine supplementation increases lifespan, through increased clearance of methionine. Restriction of dietary methionine, an essential amino acid, extends lifespan much in the same way that calorie restriction does so; some scientists argue that calorie restriction works that way precisely because it restricts methionine. The amount of glycine fed to those rats with increased lifespan was approximately 3 to 6 times the amount fed to controls, which may be doable in humans. A few grams of glycine daily might do the trick and act to mimic methionine restriction.

Could the mechanism of the increased dietary glycine that caused greater lifespan be that it made the rats' mitochondria more youthful? Yes, it could be. Methionine restriction results in much better mitochondrial function, so that's probably what the glycine is doing, since increased glycine is a methionine restriction mimetic.[88]

Glycine can also increase glutathione in mitochondria, and since glutathione is the cells' and the mitochondria's main internal antioxidant, this protects them from oxidative damage and keeps them in a youthful state. Glutathione is made from three amino acids, one of which is glycine, and if glycine is in short supply inside the mitochondria, then there will be less glutathione there. Methionine restriction also increases mitochondrial glutathione levels.

The authors of the paper themselves suggest that glycine supplementation could decrease or reverse aging. Although much more work will be needed, the study may open up a new avenue in potential anti-aging and life extension treatments.

Glycine can help relieve oxidative stress, an important component of aging. Oxidative stress occurs when the body's own internal antioxidant system, the most important element of which is glutathione, becomes depleted. Glycine is one of the components of glutathione, the other two being glutamine and cysteine. In a group of elderly people, the concentrations of glycine, cysteine, and glutathione in red blood cells were markedly lower than in younger people. Supplemental glycine and cysteine for two weeks fully restored glutathione.[89]

Glycine also improves sleep quality when ingested at 3 grams before bedtime.[90] Since other sleep medications have all manner of unwanted side effects, may be addictive, and may increase death rates, glycine makes a good choice of supplement for improved sleep.

Some foods, such as gelatin and bone broth, contain fairly high amounts of glycine, but if you want glycine for the uses we've discussed above, then a supplement may be needed. Note that in very large amounts, glycine may be toxic, but appears to be safe at the low amounts discussed here, though full toxicity studies have not been done.

Glycine Summary

- Glycine, normally found in food, may improve mitochondrial function
- It may mimic the potent lifespan-extension method of methionine restriction
- Glycine may improve sleep quality

Melatonin

Melatonin is a hormone produced by the pineal gland in the brain that helps regulate sleep. Light and dark strongly switch melatonin production off and on, respectively. Melatonin as a supplement can be used to treat insomnia. Aging tends to decrease the production of melatonin, which may partially explain increasing insomnia with age.

Melatonin also has strong neuroprotective properties, and it extends lifespan and decreases cancer in mice.[91]

In older people with insomnia, a sustained-release formula of melatonin, 2 mg, significantly improved sleep, and there appeared to be no rebound insomnia or withdrawal effects; incidence of adverse effects was low and side effects were minor.[92] A review of melatonin studies found that melatonin may not be effective in "treating most primary sleep disorders with short-term use (4 weeks or less); however, additional large-scale RCTs [randomized controlled trials] are needed before firm conclusions can be drawn." It went on to state that melatonin may be effective against "delayed sleep phase syndrome", i.e. inability to get to sleep until late, and "is safe with short-term use (3 months or less)."[93]

Be aware that use of melatonin can cause morning grogginess. Its use at low doses as a sleep aid, however, appears to be far safer than prescription or over-the-counter sleep aids.

Anecdotally, my own experience with melatonin has been less than positive. I've felt quite intense grogginess the morning after using it, so much so that I had to stop using it, as I simply couldn't get anything done in the morning. Other users I've spoken with have not had this problem. The scientific literature is a mixed bag regarding effectiveness, although its safety in short-term use and at low doses seems agreed upon.

The fact that it extends lifespan in animals speaks to its safety as well as its anti-aging properties. It increases antioxidant defense mechanisms and may prevent cancer. Many people appear to be taking melatonin expressly to fight aging.

If desired for sleep, melatonin should be started at the lowest dose possible to avoid side effects. The National Sleep Foundation, an advocacy group, recommends an adult dose starting at 200 μg (two tenths of a milligram), and then increasing that as needed.[94]

Melatonin and light exposure

As the absence of light stimulates the release of melatonin, a word on light exposure and sleep is in order. Exposure to bright light at night disrupts sleep by disrupting melatonin production, and if you need melatonin to sleep, it's possible that in reality all you need to do is reduce your light exposure.

Not only does light at night disrupt melatonin, but light in the evening does also. Exposure to light in the bedroom can lower melatonin production *by half*. Light in the blue range of the spectrum appears to be doing most of the harm here.

There are a number of things you can do about light in the evening and night if you have sleep problems. Keep room lights low in the evening for starters.

We increasingly use computers, including tablets and phones, at all hours, and they emit strong light in the blue wavelength range, disrupting sleep. There are a number of computer programs that both dim the light from computer screens and change the color composition so that the light contains less blue. These programs are a must for people who use their computers at night. These programs include f.lux (for Windows) and Twilight for Android. Word is getting out, as Kindle Fire tablets now have a built-in program, Blue Shade.

There remains the problem of watching television at night, as they cause the same light problems. For this, you can use a pair of blue-blocking safety glasses, which are cheap and solve the problem. You might feel a bit weird wearing yellow glasses around your house, but it's worth it if you get better sleep out of it.

Using the same considerations as above, morning exposure to bright, full-spectrum light, i.e. the sun, helps entrain circadian rhythms, making for better health. There's a great deal of evidence that exposure to bright light in the morning helps relieve depression. A simple way to get more morning light is merely not wearing sunglasses. If you commute to work, for example, don't wear sunglasses during your drive (or walk if you're so fortunate, bus ride, etc.). I like to go for a walk in the morning, and I make it a practice never to wear sunglasses while doing so.

If you live in a place where there's little morning sunlight, such as in the north and in the winter, artificial light sources that emit full-spectrum bright light are available (and relatively inexpensive). You can sit in front of one for 30 minutes or so in the morning and get bright light exposure; this practice can relieve depression when done properly and for the correct duration. People with a tendency to mania should not use bright light exposure, however, as light may exacerbate that condition.

Melatonin Summary

- The brain hormone melatonin promotes sleep

- It's extended lifespan in animals
- Light at night disrupts the production of melatonin
- It may cause morning grogginess and should only be used in minimal doses
- Natural or artificial bright light in the morning can improve circadian rhythms

Quercetin

Many of the substances discussed in this section overlap in their effects, perhaps mainly by activating AMPK, the master cellular energy sensor, and thus partly mimic calorie restriction. For example, berberine, metformin, green tea, resveratrol, and curcumin all do this, so there's probably little need to take more than one or two of them, depending on your needs and the other effects of these substances. It's not known how much a combination of these substances might be overdoing it, or what the effects of that might be, so you should tread carefully when deciding which combination, if any, to use.

Quercetin is another plant-derived substance that has similar effects, and it's worth discussing here for the sake of completeness.

Senescent cells drive aging. Senescent cells are those which have reached the end of their road, having divided many times and reached the limit of their life. Unfortunately, they don't die, but enter a stage of senescence in which they emit inflammatory molecules and generally make life miserable for their neighboring cells. They put the entire body into an inflammatory state.

How much of the phenotype of old age is due to senescent cells is not known, but most scientists in this field consider them very important. If we could get rid of senescent cells, animals, including humans, might lose many of the characteristics of old age and might literally become younger. Even if senescent cells comprise only 10 to 15% of all cells, that makes a big difference, and even partially eliminating them could mean a much healthier organism.

Recently, scientists tested a combination of two substances, quercetin and dasatinib (the latter an anti-cancer drug) for their ability to eliminate senescent cells in old mice.[95] The combination was effective at eliminating mouse senescent embryonic fibroblasts, and dasatinib alone more effective at eliminating senescent human fat cells, but of interest, quercetin was more effective at eliminating senescent human endothelial cells.

The lowering of senescent cell burden in old mice led to improved cardiac function 5 days after a single dose. In mice subject to irradiation treatment of one leg to promote cellular senescence, one dose of the drug combination led to improved exercise capacity for at least 7 months after a single dose.

The results of this experiment suggest that quercetin could eliminate some senescent cells in humans. The dose of quercetin used on the mice was 50 mg per kg of bodyweight. Using a standard algorithm to translate that dose to humans arrives at a human dose, for a 70-kg man, of approximately 300 mg. (Dose per unit of bodyweight is divided by 12 to account for the difference in metabolism between mice and men.)

Quercetin is present in food at an estimated 5-40 mg daily. Human studies have shown no adverse effects of one month of quercetin at 500 mg twice daily, but higher doses,

3.5 grams a day, have shown renal toxicity.[96] However, an older study found that quercetin shortened the lifespan of mice, and another found that it had no effect on mouse lifespan.[97] In the context of senescent cells, these results may make sense: enough toxicity to eliminate senescent cells, not enough for overall toxicity.

Quercetin, besides it's direct (putative) anti-aging effect on senescent cells, may have effects against cardiovascular disease and cancer.

A study that was published as this book is being written showed the tremendous power of eliminating senescent cells. (This study did not use quercetin.)[98] Mice became remarkably younger looking and ran up to 350% greater distance daily than those not treated. Truly this could be a fountain of youth if results are replicated in humans, and some observers expect that this will happen soon.

Quercetin Summary

- Quercetin is a plant product that affects biology similarly to resveratrol, curcumin, and others
- Quercetin may eliminate senescent cells
- Most of the prospects for quercetin are speculative, although it appears to have activity against heart disease and cancer
- High doses have a potential for toxicity

N-Acetylcysteine

N-acetylcysteine (NAC) is sometimes known as a pro-drug, meaning that it metabolizes to something else inside the body, and this metabolite exerts the physiological effect. NAC becomes the amino acid cysteine, which is an essential amino acid, a required nutrient. (Cysteine is sometimes termed "conditionally essential", since the body can make it from another amino acid, methionine, but not always in sufficient quantities.) Amino acids, of which cysteine is one, are the constituents of proteins, which are in turn components of virtually all foods, and are found in large amounts especially in animal products such as meat, eggs, and dairy.

When NAC is ingested, cells take it up rapidly, the acetyl group is removed, and the active ingredient, cysteine, remains. So then, why wouldn't you just take cysteine?

Cysteine is a sulfur amino acid, and easily oxidized, which makes taking it as a supplement non-optimal. By adding the acetyl group to cysteine, the molecule becomes much more stable, storable, and suitable for use as a supplement.

Cysteine is an important constituent of the molecule glutathione.

Antioxidants are molecules in food that capture free radicals inside cells, detoxify them, and prevent oxidative damage. Controlling free radicals is important, and therefore the body has not left this to the chance ingestion of certain foods, but has evolved its own antioxidant system. The system includes enzymes such as catalase and superoxide dismutase, and the small molecule, glutathione. Glutathione is the most abundant — and therefore, important — component of the body's antioxidant system.

Three amino acids, glycine, glutamine, and cysteine, make up glutathione. Of these three, glycine and glutamine are non-essential amino acids made by the body, which usually has all it needs. Cysteine, however, may not always be available and has therefore been termed the "rate-limiting" amino acid in glutathione synthesis.

In simple terms, not enough cysteine, then not enough glutathione.

Levels of glutathione decline in disease and aging.[99] Cells use glutathione to detoxify free radicals, and it must then must be replaced or recycled. When cells' metabolic machinery generates large enough amounts of free radicals occur under stressful conditions and overpower the internal antioxidant system's capacity, glutathione is depleted and a state of oxidative stress exists. These stressful conditions include infection, diabetes, cancer, aging, and even exercise.

By supplying cysteine in the form of NAC, glutathione can be replenished and oxidative stress reduced or eliminated. This is the source of the health benefits of NAC.

The glutathione system is considered a target of therapy in a number of neuroimmune disorders, including depression and chronic fatigue.[100]

Oxidative stress also causes disruption of important hormonal and other cellular signals, since these signals depend on molecular shape and interaction, and these in turn depend on pH and the redox status of the cellular milieu. The body doesn't function optimally in oxidative stress.

NAC has been tested in:

- Psychiatric illness
- Chronic fatigue

- Influenza
- Heavy metal chelation
- Aging

NAC replenishes glutathione, including in the brain, and this is likely its mechanism of action in various psychiatric illnesses.

Bipolar depression: An open-label trial of NAC in patients with bipolar depression yielded "a robust decrement in depression scores". The patients took 1 gram NAC, twice a day, and this was as "a maintenance treatment for bipolar disorder."[101]

Addiction: NAC has been studied for its effects in cocaine, marijuana, and nicotine addiction, with varying success, and studies are ongoing.[102]

NAC in chronic fatigue: NAC may be useful in treating chronic fatigue. In chronic fatigue, oxidative damage to DNA is higher than in controls, which indicates the presence of oxidative stress.[103] It's been speculated that competition between the immune system and muscle for glutathione precursors such as cysteine favors the immune system.[104] When that happens, muscles become depleted of glutathione and cannot function properly, leading to fatigue and myalgia. A number of studies have found depleted levels of glutathione in chronic fatigue syndrome, and n-acetylcysteine results in improvement of symptoms.[105]

Michael Maes, the biological psychiatrist who's done a great deal of research on chronic fatigue, found that normalization of leaky gut in chronic fatigue patients resulted in clinical improvement.[106] Among the supplements that Maes says improve gut barrier function are glutamine, zinc, and n-acetylcysteine.

One of the more remarkable studies on NAC has been in the prevention of influenza. A total of 262 people, 78% of them over 65 years of age, and most of them suffering from a chronic illness, were randomized to 600 mg NAC twice a day for 6 months, or placebo. Frequency of seroconversion, that is, the development of antibodies to a particular strain of flu virus, was about the same in either NAC or placebo groups. But only 25% of the NAC group who were infected developed symptoms, as opposed to 79% of the placebo group.[107] NAC also prevents the replication of the flu virus in cell culture.

In people with chronic bronchitis, NAC at a dose of 300 mg, twice a day, dramatically reduced the number of sick days.[108]

NAC chelates heavy metals, such as methylmercury, lead, and cadmium.[109] Heavy metals are seriously toxic and can lead to heart disease and other illnesses.

NAC can increase time to fatigue in endurance exercise.[110] In cyclists who took 1200 mg daily of NAC for 9 days, sprint performance time was improved and oxidative damage was decreased.[111] NAC increases fat oxidation during exercise and lowers lactate levels, but may decrease power output.[112]

NAC could function as an antioxidant, and prevent the health-promoting effects of exercise. However, taking NAC after exercise could promote better recovery, since exercise depletes glutathione. In general, though, the damage caused by exercise is part and parcel of its effect on improving performance and health. Whether NAC ultimately improves or decreases exercise performance over the long run remains unknown. NAC is not a banned substance in sports, and if it worked as well as suggested, it probably would be.

Aging has been characterized as a cysteine-deficiency syndrome.[113] Oxidative stress, and consequent lower glutathione levels, affect each other in a vicious cycle. Inflammation increases, and autophagy decreases.

A double-blind study in frail elderly people found that NAC doubled leg extension strength during a 6-week exercise program, and those taking placebo had *zero* increase in strength.[114] TNF-alpha, an inflammatory cytokine, decreased. Based on this, NAC could be quite useful in the frail elderly to help get them less frail and improve their quality of life.

Is NAC safe?

NAC is controversial regarding safety. A few years ago, a study found that mice that were given NAC developed pulmonary arterial hypertension, a serious condition that can be fatal in humans. Dr. Joseph Mercola, a trustworthy source whose opinions are worth heeding, states that NAC "could cause you loads of trouble".[115] He says that "a little is probably OK – even good for you... However, using large quantities is probably not good for you.... If used therapeutically it should be used in low doses for 'prevention'." He states that cancer patients should *not* use it.

A review paper on the use of NAC in psychiatry states, "Some adverse events, such as pulmonary hypertension are reported in very high-dose animal studies, but have not been seen in human studies."[116]

Julius Goepp, M.D., writing in Life Extension magazine, says, "There have been no further publications supporting this one-time observation made in an animal model using doses 10-20 times those suggested for long-term human supplementation. No human study has uncovered any evidence for a similar effect in humans. By contrast, there have been numerous studies demonstrating human benefit from NAC supplementation at moderate doses (1,200-1,800 mg per day) over the course of nearly 4 decades."[117]

A review paper, "N-acetylcysteine – a safe antidote for cysteine/glutathione deficiency" states, "Oral administration of NAC [is] a safe well-tolerated drug with no clinically significant adverse effects."[118]

Given the expert opinions cited above, I'm inclined to be cautious about NAC.

In reality, NAC is merely a delivery system for an amino acid, cysteine. Since whey protein is both high in cysteine and generally a high-quality protein, NAC may be merely a proxy for better dietary protein. In other words, if the people with bipolar, chronic fatigue, flu, etc., had had a greater intake of high quality protein, would they even need NAC? Would they have those disorders in the first place?

I've seen people with chronic fatigue who have a green smoothie and a banana for breakfast. That kind of eating, lauded in some places as healthy, has so little protein that you're almost guaranteed to feel lousy if you eat that way all the time.

Likewise for the elderly people with "cysteine deficiency". Maybe if they ate a better diet with meat and eggs and cheese instead of a plate of spaghetti or a can of Ensure or whatever it is they eat, they wouldn't need extra cysteine.

That, however, is speculation. But the fact remains that you can replenish cysteine and thus glutathione with whey protein, and that, we know, is completely safe.

Theanine for anxiety

Theanine (or L-theanine) is an amino acid found almost exclusively in the tea plant, *Camellia sinensis*, and therefore is contained in tea. It is generally considered safe in humans, and it extends lifespan in the worm *C. elegans*.[119] Theanine promotes attention, that is, it's a kind of nootropic, and it may have favorable effects on body weight and blood pressure.

Theanine can reduce anxiety and induce relaxation without causing drowsiness, and that is its main source of interest as a supplement.[120] A dose of from 50 to 200 mg induces alpha brain waves within 40 minutes. In rats that are spontaneously hypertensive, theanine reduces blood pressure.

In patients with schizophrenia, theanine at 200 mg, twice a day, and added to the patients' ongoing anti-psychotic medication, significantly relieved anxiety, with effects "from modest to moderate".[121] "L-Theanine was found to be a safe and well-tolerated medication."

Theanine appears to be exceptionally non-toxic; rats treated with 4000 milligrams per kilogram of body weight, a very high dose indeed, showed no adverse effects, and no higher doses were tested.[122] The U.S. FDA lists theanine as GRAS (Generally Recognized As Safe).[123] (On the other hand, prescription anti-anxiety drugs are not safe, and can lead to overdose, addiction, and accidents.) Contrary to expectations, a cup of black tea has more theanine, 24 mg, than green tea, at 8 mg.[124]

Optimal doses are not known with any certainty, but most clinical studies have used from 50 to 200 mg.

Theanine is probably the best over-the-counter anti-anxiety supplement around.

Ketone Supplements

When you eat a very low carbohydrate diet, or fast for more than about 16 hours, the body produces ketones. Ketones (often referred to as ketone bodies) are made in the liver from fatty acids that have left the fat cells, and these ketones partially substitute for blood glucose, since many cells in the body can use them in place of glucose.

Ketones have a number of therapeutic uses, most prominently in the treatment of intractable epilepsy, in which very low carbohydrate diets can be more effective than drugs in some cases. A low-carbohydrate, ketogenic (ketone-producing) diet is also a solid weight-loss diet.

Low-carbohydrate diets and fasting affect several biochemical pathways, notably insulin, which it decreases, and that's one source of their benefits.

Another source of their benefits is ketones themselves, and ketones now come in a can (or bottle or bag). Taking a ketone supplement could give you many of the benefits of low-carb and fasting without actually, you know, eating low-carb or fasting.

Ketone supplements may modestly increase athletic performance, although more evidence is needed.[125] Naturally, professional cyclists aren't waiting for more evidence and use of ketone supplements is allegedly widespread among them.

Ketone supplements also promote longevity.[126] The main ketone body, beta hydroxybutyrate (BHB), mimics the lifespan extending effects of calorie restriction, i.e. it's a calorie restriction mimetic. Scientists have developed numerous theories about how calorie restriction promotes longevity, but one reliably reproduced effect of CR across all species is the production of ketone bodies, including BHB. Some scientists believe that BHB will also extend lifespan in humans.

Ketone supplements can suppress hunger without raising blood glucose or insulin. When animals are given a ketone supplement, their glucose and insulin levels drop. Ketone supplements also lead to lower body weight in rats. I've tried them myself, and my appetite disappeared when I took them.

Several ketone supplements are available, such as KetoCaNa, InstaKetones, and Pruvit Keto//os. The drawback is that they're expensive, at $2 or more a serving. But they work, so it depends on whether that's worth it to you. Using MCT oil may give many of the benefits but at a lower price. I should add that these ketone supplements are not the same as so-called "raspberry ketones", a bogus weight-loss product.

Cheap Anti-Aging Supplements

There are a number of proprietary and relatively expensive supplements marketed as having anti-aging activity. The two that are best-known are Protandim and Longevinex. In reality, you don't need to spend a lot of money to get the benefits of supplements like these.

135

The company that sells Protandim bills it as "The Nrf2 Synergizer", since it up-regulates the cellular stress defense mechanisms via the Nrf2 (nuclear erythroid factor 2) system, a master regulator of antioxidant defenses. Activated Nrf2 produces the phase 2 enzymes: catalase, superoxide dismutase, and various enzymes that catalyze metabolism of xenobiotics, including drugs. Notably included in the phase 2 group is ferritin, which captures free iron and prevents it from doing damage. These enzymes prevent oxidative stress, cancer, and other maladies of aging.

Contact with foreign molecules that need detoxifying activates Nrf2. Hence this system involves hormesis, in which low doses of a toxin or other input such as exercise or fasting produce beneficial health effects.

The ingredients in Protandim promote hormesis. It's a proprietary blend of a total of 675 mg of extracts of milk thistle, bacopa, ashwaghanda, turmeric (i.e. curcumin), and green tea. Of these, I occasionally take curcumin and drink green tea, giving me two out of five of the ingredients already.

Protandim retails online for just under $35 for 30 capsules, or a one-month supply. Pricey, if you plan to take it for any extended time.

The other supplement, Longevinex, claims to be designed to mimic calorie restriction, the robust life extension intervention. (Many of the benefits and few of the downsides of calorie restriction can be obtained through intermittent fasting.)

The ingredients of a capsule of Longevinex are vitamin D3 (1000 IU), and 244 mg of a proprietary blend of resveratrol (at 100 mg per capsule), unknown quantities of inositol hexaphosphate (IP6), quercetin, chlorogenic acid, green tea extract, and "nucleotides".

Longevinex retails for about the same price as Protandim, or about $34 for a 30-day supply. Their new product, Advantage, retails for $50 a month.

Let's say I wanted to both activate my Nrf2 system and mimic calorie restriction using these premium products. That could cost me a minimum of $70 a month, or $840 a year. Also, keep in mind that most people buying these products don't know much or even anything about their ingredients, and probably think of these products as unique or magical. While the ingredients have sound scientific backing, it's not necessary to buy these particular products to get the ingredients.

As it happens, in my rotation of supplements I have curcumin, IP6, vitamin D, and resveratrol, and I drink tea, providing many of the ingredients of both of these. Chlorogenic acid, an ingredient of Longevinex, is found abundantly in coffee, and may provide many of its benefits. And I do drink coffee.

Many of these are cheap. IP6 in bulk is about $20 for 250 grams (over half a pound); at 500 mg a day, that will last 500 days. Green tea is cheap at a few cents for a cup. Curcumin is the only one that's relatively expensive, but even here, at about $26 for 120 capsules, and if not taken every day, it will last quite a while.

It's worth noting that neither proprietary supplement contains aspirin, which not only may be one of the most potent anti-aging drugs available, but is literally the world's cheapest drug.

Expensive, proprietary anti-aging supplements can easily be, if not duplicated, at least reasonably imitated with cheap OTC, generic supplements.

It's possible that we wouldn't get all of the benefits of Protandim and Longevinex because some of the ingredients are missing. I don't take milk thistle, ashwaghanda, bacopa, or quercetin.

But is it likely we're missing any of the benefits? That seems highly doubtful to me.

For one thing, I already practice an intervention that mimics calorie restriction, namely intermittent fasting. I also exercise, another hormetic process.

Maybe more importantly, I drink coffee, tea, and red wine, and eat chocolate, which provide high levels of dietary polyphenols and greatly lower disease risk. The other ingredients in the two proprietary supplements would be unlikely to add much of value to what I already do.

I also eat vegetables, especially broccoli, onions, peppers, and the like, which strongly up-regulate the Nrf2 system. Broccoli and other cruciferous vegetables are known to have a strong anti-cancer effect. Again, given my intake of these and other dietary components high in hormetic constituents – like coffee, tea, chocolate, and red wine – it's doubtful that Protandim and/or Longevinex would add in any appreciable way to the health benefits I already get from both supplements, food, and lifestyle.

So, instead of spending big bucks on Protandim and Longevinex, consider doing it the cheap way. It will likely provide more and better anti-aging effects anyway.

Polyphenols: How Much Is Too Much?

Several of the supplements in this section, including resveratrol, black and green tea, curcumin, quercetin, and berberine, are polyphenols, a class of chemicals found in plants. In addition, coffee, black tea, chocolate, and red wine contain relatively large amounts of these phytochemicals. If you consume these foods/beverages and also supplement, is it possible to get too many polyphenols to be compatible with good health?

Consumption of polyphenols is robustly associated with better health and lower death rates and a 46% reduction in cardiovascular disease risk.[127],[128] These studies were based on the polyphenol content of foods, such as coffee, fruits and vegetables, etc., as well as a spot urine test for polyphenols, but not supplement use. The highest intakes of polyphenols, that is, those associated with the lowest death rates, averaged about 1235 mg a day.

To get a handle on this, it helps to know the polyphenol content of some common food items, notably those high in them as we've discussed. I've listed the total polyphenol content, by serving, in the following, calculated from the amount in 100 grams or in 100 ml from "Identification of the 100 richest dietary sources of polyphenols: an application of the Phenol-Explorer database".[129]

- Dark chocolate: ~500 mg
- Coffee: ~300 mg
- Black tea: ~150 mg
- Green tea: ~120 mg
- Red wine: ~150 mg

Someone who drinks two regular-size (6-ounce) cups of coffee daily, eats a serving of dark chocolate, and has two glasses of red wine (for example), will have a polyphenol intake of around 1400 mg. (Rough calculation.) That's about the level seen in the highest category of polyphenol consumption and the category with the lowest death rates. Using some different assumptions, it would appear to be relatively easy to get total daily polyphenol uptake into the several-thousand-milligram daily range. In fact, a 20-ounce coffee of the kind sold in chain coffee shops may alone have 1200 mg of polyphenols.

For comparison, some of the doses of supplements we've discussed, such as berberine and curcumin, are 500 mg. Resveratrol suggested doses are lower, at 100 mg or less.

Could you get too many polyphenols, or is there even such a thing as too many?

Hormesis and polyphenols

Unfortunately, the answer is not known. It may or may not follow that, because those who consumed 1250 mg of polyphenols a day had the lowest death rates, those who consumed 2500 mg a day have even lower death rates. Maybe they do, maybe they don't. A point of diminishing returns likely exists somewhere. Furthermore, not all polyphenols are the same and some have greater effects than others and/or use different mechanisms of action, so adding them into all one basket for purposes of calculating total intake may be of limited value.

Stilbenes and lignans

The study that found 37% lower death rates also reported, "Among the polyphenol subclasses, stilbenes and lignans were significantly associated with reduced all-cause mortality [HR 0.48 and 0.60, respectively], with no significant associations apparent in the rest (flavonoids or phenolic acids)."

If polyphenols cause lower death rates (that is, it's not mere association), then only certain classes of them count for much.

The two classes of polyphenols that mattered were stilbenes, which include resveratrol, pterostilbene, and other compounds in grapes, wine, and cocoa; and lignans, the richest source of which is flaxseed.

Since polyphenols most likely work through hormesis, the process by which low doses of toxins or stressors produce beneficial health effects, it follows that at some dosage, polyphenols may be overtly toxic, and damage health.

The point I wish to make is to be aware of what you're taking and not to overdo it. Don't indiscriminately take large amounts of different polyphenol supplements in the quest for ever better health, especially if you already drink coffee, tea, and wine, and eat chocolate. Not to mention if you eat berries, another source of large amounts of polyphenols, or if you cover your food with cloves – just kidding, but that's the number one food for polyphenols.

Although we don't know at what, if any, level that polyphenols become a problem, and overt toxicity in animals seems to occur only at very high doses, if you tally up your polyphenol intake, including supplements, and find it at, say, over a couple thousand milligrams daily, I would consider cutting back. These considerations may not apply to those with special health needs, such as someone taking berberine several times a day for blood sugar control, but such people should have cleared their use of supplements with their doctor first.

Supplement Timing

The time at which you take a particular supplement can make a difference in its effects. Usually the effects are not pronounced, but certain considerations may make taking a supplement at one time of the day rather than another better.

For example, I often practice *intermittent fasting*, which means going without food for 16 hours or more, usually from dinner in the evening until about noon the next day. One of the main benefits of intermittent fasting lies in the promotion of autophagy, the cellular self-cleansing process that rids cells of junk. Eating strongly decreases, and fasting strongly increases, the process of autophagy; the presence of nutrients (i.e. food, especially protein and carbohydrates) is the main factor in whether autophagy takes place.

Some people advocate fasting along with taking BCAAs and/or whey protein, in order to help preserve muscle mass while losing fat. The practice of using BCAAs or whey for this is perfectly acceptable, and will likely help you retain muscle. However, BCAAs and/or protein will both completely shut down autophagy; if you practice intermittent fasting for anti-aging purposes, to promote the process of autophagy, taking BCAAs/protein is counter-productive. Therefore, those are supplements to avoid during fasting, unless your fasting is strictly for the purpose of weight loss; take them (if desired) during the fed state, that period of several hours immediately during and following a meal.

Some supplements promote autophagy, and these include resveratrol and berberine. Taking them in the fasted state can boost autophagy levels beyond what is seen in fasting, and thus may make a session of intermittent fasting even more of an anti-aging intervention.

Vitamins C and E interfere with and blunt the healthful effects of exercise; while we've cautioned against taking too much of either of these supplements, there may be reasons to take them, for instance if you find yourself coming down with colds more often than you could reasonably expect. If you do decide to take vitamins C or E, do not take them around your exercise sessions, either before or after. How long the intervals should be between taking one of these vitamins and your exercise is difficult to say, but several hours is a reasonable guess, since in that time much of the vitamin would be gone from the bloodstream and taken up by cells. At high doses, however (1000 mg for C, 250 mg for E), even taking them away from exercise may still blunt exercise effects.

There are anecdotal reports of vitamin D, when taken in the evening, interfering with sleep. I know of no research that backs up this claim, but logically it makes some sense, since the action of the sun on the skin produces vitamin D, and thus that may be connected to circadian rhythms and sleep. Since to me it's no big deal when I take vitamin D, when I do take it, I do so in the morning.

On the other side of the equation, magnesium has a relaxing effect and can improve sleep. I can always use help with my sleep, so I take my magnesium at bedtime.

Some supplements, such as curcumin, are poorly absorbed from the gut, and taking them with a high-fat meal improves absorption.

Inositol hexaphosphate (IP6) chelates iron and other metals, and if taken with food, the presence of metals in the food effectively neutralizes IP6. It should be taken on an empty stomach.

Quick Guide to Supplement Timing

If any of these supplements are desired, do the following:

- BCAAs and/or whey or other protein, during the fed state
- Resveratrol and berberine boost autophagy in the fasted state
- Vitamins C and E, away from exercise
- Vitamin D, in the morning
- Magnesium, if sleep improvement needed, in the evening
- Curcumin, with food
- IP6, on an empty stomach

Ray Kurzweil's supplement stack, and why it's probably the wrong approach

Ray Kurzweil (b. 1948), is a noted computer scientist, futurist, and author of a number of books, most notably *The Singularity Is Near*, in which he states his case for a scenario of the future so technologically advanced that it's literally beyond imagination. In part, according to him, the singularity will result in humans living longer than ever, perhaps hundreds or thousands of years; in order to reach that point in which technology allows such extended human lifespans, we must practice anti-aging regimens now. And Kurzweil does this. He allegedly takes as many as 77 different supplements for anti-aging and health purposes.[130] Here's a partial list:

- Comprehensive multi-vitamin, coenzyme Q10, grapeseed extract, resveratrol, bilberry extract, lycopene, silymarine, linoleic acid, lecithin, n-acetylcysteine, garlic, l-carnitine, pyrodoxal-5-phosphate [a form of vitamin B6], echinacea, B12 shots.
- Chromium, metformin, Gymnema sylvestra.
- Policosanol, gugulipid, plant sterols, niacin, oat bran, grapefruit powder, psyllium, lecithin, Lipitor [a statin].
- Arginine, TMG, choline.
- Aspirin, lumbrokinase.
- EPA/DHA, curcumin.
- Folic acid, B6.
- EDTA, DMPS.
- Intravenous glutathione
- Intravenous phosphatidylcholine
- PtC, DHEA, Testosterone, l-3-C, chrysin, nettle, ginger.
- Saw palmetto complex
- L-theanine, beta-sitosterol, Phosphatidylserine, Green tea extract.
- GABA, melatonin, glycerylphosphatidylcholine, nextrutine, quercertin.
- Lutein, bilberry extract.

- Antioxidant skin creams.
- Betaine HCL, pepsin, gentian root, peppermint, Acidophilus bifodobacter, fructooligosaccharides [prebiotics], fish proteins, l-glutamine, n-acetyl-d-glucosamine.
- N-acetyl-carnitine, carnosine, quercertin, alpha lipoic acid

While Kurzweil's supplement regimen allegedly costs thousands of dollars a day, he can probably afford it. The real questions that arise are:

- Do you need to take so many supplements for optimal anti-aging?

- Could Kurzweil be overdoing it, and instead of counteracting aging, be promoting it?

To answer these questions, we need to know what they do.

On the list, several are polyphenols, and as we saw in the section on too many polyphenols, it's possible he could be taking too much and/or the supplements overlap in mechanisms and they're not all necessary. Doses are not listed in the sources I've seen, but in that group, grape seed extract, resveratrol, curcumin, green tea extract, and quercetin are all polyphenols and have many overlapping effects. Furthermore, Kurzweil eats a high-polyphenol diet, reportedly including raspberries, blackberries, dark chocolate, and green tea. If that's typical for his food, Kurzweil may have a polyphenol intake, including supplements, of many thousands of milligrams daily. There's a tremendous lack of knowledge whether that amount of polyphenols is either necessary for health, or even harmful to health. Kurzweil wants to live longer to take advantage of future anti-aging medicine and technology, which implies that he wants either a guarantee or a reasonable shot that his regimen will work. But there could be a good chance that his regimen is harmful, tipping on to the far side of the hormetic J-curve into toxicity.

Kurzweil also takes a statin drug, Lipitor, which probably does more harm than good. His cholesterol is reportedly around 100 mg/dl, a value so low that it endangers his health. Higher cholesterol is associated with longer life.[131] Low cholesterol, below 160 mg/dl, is associated with violence, suicide, and cancer.[132] Besides lower cholesterol, statins have all kinds of nasty side effects, such as muscle pain and memory loss, which isn't surprising, since cholesterol is a necessary and vital component of cell membranes. Statins aren't even very effective at preventing heart attacks. In this matter, Kurzweil adheres to some very old-style thinking on the cause of cardiovascular disease; insulin resistance likely plays a huge role, and lowering cholesterol does little if anything.

Kurzweil doesn't appear to take magnesium or zinc. Both are powerfully involved in anti-aging and are arguably much more important than many of the other supplements he takes.

You have to get your theories of aging right in order to effectively fight aging. Science has found a number of good theories and measures as to what promotes aging or counteracts it; calorie restriction stands, for now, as the archetype of an anti-aging intervention. Fewer calories, or substances that mimic the physiological processes that occur with fewer calories, offer the best shot at counteracting aging. Given our relative paucity of knowledge on the realities of preventing or reversing aging, however, it doesn't make much sense to use a shotgun approach like Kurzweil has, in my estimation. As we've noted, some of these may be counterproductive or harmful. Just as in medicine, the first objective in fighting aging should be to do no harm.

We could mention a few more items on Kurzweil's list that might do harm. A multivitamin may contain iron, copper, and calcium, which are on my list of supplements not to take. He does take aspirin, in his case likely a good thing, but I won't bore the reader by going through the entire list. Many of them strike me as ineffective at best.

The Pareto principle states that 20% of inputs cause 80% of outputs. Using this principle, it stands that each additional supplement does not add equally to the desired outcome, which is anti-aging and long life. So, even if you think Kurzweil's approach is the way to go, if you found the top dozen or so supplements, you'd be effectively duplicating the longevity effect, even if that involves quite a bit of guesswork. Here are what I believe to be the most effective supplements on the list:

- Grape seed extract
- Resveratrol
- Metformin (a prescription drug)
- Aspirin
- Curcumin
- Melatonin
- Green tea (though I'd just drink it, not take the extract)
- EPA/DHA (omega-3 fatty acids)

I have difficulty getting too excited about anything else on the list. Hopefully, Kurzweil also practices intermittent fasting and strength training, key interventions which I discussed in my book *Stop the Clock: The Optimal Anti-Aging Strategy*. Those interventions could make much more of a difference than at least half the supplements he takes, in my estimation.

Some supplements truly fight aging, but figuring out which ones they are from a long list isn't always easy. Most – maybe all – of the supplements on Kurzweil's list are backed by science, but have only a few animal experiments to their credit. Not all of them by any means have been shown to prolong lifespan in experimental animals. Besides, just because a supplement affects a certain physiological parameter doesn't mean that it works via a unique biochemical mechanism. Many of the supplements on his list likely do the same things, so many of the supplements are superfluous. They either chelate iron, deactivate mTOR, increase insulin sensitivity, or all of these at once.

One of the keys to living a long life is to maintain insulin sensitivity, as the famous experiments of Cynthia Kenyon have shown. While supplements like metformin or curcumin can help maintain insulin sensitivity, the most effective tools for that are exercise, especially strength training, and avoidance of sugar, refined carbohydrates, and industrial seed oils. Becoming or remaining lean and muscular potently prevents insulin resistance, so that's a requirement for long life. Other interventions include keeping iron levels in the low normal range, intermittent fasting for maintaining autophagy at youthful levels, along with other key lifestyle factors like a good social life with lots of friends, a decent marriage, staying active, even going to church. Supplements can be important, and I wouldn't have written an entire book about them if they weren't, but don't count on them alone to prolong your life. Neglect of the other factors would likely negate any advantage you get from them.

Long Life – Key Points

- Calorie restriction (CR) is the archetype for the way in which most supplements can extend life
- Resveratrol mimics CR
- Curcumin and berberine activate AMPK
- Tea is associated with longer life, and both black and green teas are probably equally effective
- Vitamins D and K fight cancer and heart disease and many are deficient in them
- Aspirin is one of the more potent life-extension drugs, but can have serious side effects
- IP6 binds and removes iron, and therefore prevents cancer
- Glycine mimics methionine restriction
- Glucosamine is associated with longer life in humans, and extends life in lab animals
- Melatonin extends lifespan and promotes sleep
- Theanine is anti-anxiety, and safer than prescription tranquilizers
- Ketone supplements could extend lifespan.

7: Skin and Hair

Good-looking skin and hair reflect underlying health, and that's why they're prominent in our assessment of someone's attractiveness. Wrinkled skin implies that a person is old and past his prime and not, therefore, in the best of health; grey hair likewise. Attractive, youthful, and healthy-looking skin and hair are of prime importance in, to use the language of evolutionary psychology, mating effort. So, to make the most of your mating opportunities, i.e. attractiveness to the opposite sex, you should maximize the attractiveness of skin and hair.

A healthy body naturally results in healthy skin and hair, but sometimes we have problems with them even when we're doing everything we can to maintain our health. Adult acne, for example, is a common problem, and everyone gets wrinkles and grey hair, so in this chapter we'll discuss some supplements (using that term broadly) that can help. A conspicuous problem in assessing which supplements or topical agents actually work is that companies that sell them often make wild claims for them. Skin and hair care is a huge business, and many products sell at exorbitant prices. Here we'll see which agents have actual scientific backing for their alleged efficacy, and whether you need to spend a fortune to get them. (Spoiler: in almost all cases, you don't.)

As with other supplements discussed in this book, a sound diet and exercise routine provides the foundation for health, and supplements (or topical agents) can provide additional help.

Acne

Acne is most associated with teenagers, but many adults have it well into middle age. I have personal experience with adult acne, an embarrassing problem. Since it is most prominent on the face and is the outward sign of infection and inflammation, it creates a stigma for those who have it, although in my experience much of the stigma is the mind of its sufferer. Through both trial and error and studying how best to deal with it, I figured out how to prevent and eliminate it.

Acne is a condition in which pores in the skin become clogged, leading to inflammation and bacterial infection.

As with so many other health problems, it's my belief that doctors look at this problem wrongly. They see it as something that needs to be treated with drugs, rather than as something that can be prevented or that is due to lifestyle factors. In their overview of acne, the American Academy of Dermatology does not mention a single lifestyle factor as being involved in acne.[1] To them, it just sort of appears, and then you need to see one of their members for expensive treatment.

Contrary to their assessment, it's not hard to see that diet and other lifestyle factors play a key role in acne.

Consider that an examination of over 1300 people, including several hundred aged 15 to 25, failed to turn up a single case of acne.[2] The subjects examined were people living a traditional lifestyle: Kitavans (in the South Pacific) and Aché (Paraguay). The authors believe that genetic factors are not paramount, since members of closely related groups develop acne when living in Westernized societies. They aptly call acne "a disease of Western civilization".

High levels of the hormone insulin are the ultimate cause of acne, they believe, and in turn that's caused by high calories, sugar, and refined carbohydrates. In addition, dairy products may be a problem for some people.

The Kitavans, with zero cases of acne, do indeed have much lower fasting insulin and glucose levels than age-matched Swedes.[3] Kitavans eat no processed foods, since there are none available to them on their remote island; staple foods are fish, coconut, and sweet potatoes. Despite what the average doctor will tell you, diet can prevent or cause acne.

Sugar. Sugar raises insulin levels, including in the skin. In addition, high blood sugar levels that come from ingesting sugar feed the bacteria, *Propionibacterium acnes*, that infects pores after they've been blocked. High amounts of sugar reliably cause acne, and should be entirely eliminated. Consider cutting way back on refined carbohydrates (anything made with flour, such as bread, pasta, pastries, etc.) too.

Caffeine. The caffeine in coffee and tea stimulates production of oil in the skin, leading to blocked pores and acne. Caffeine is probably not as strong a cause of acne as sugar, but if you consume large amounts of it and have acne, cutting back will likely help. Note that many people put milk and sugar in their coffee and tea also, which exacerbates its acne-producing effect. Also note that chocolate has caffeine and other related stimulants like theobromine, and is usually loaded with sugar. Chocolate has long been fingered as a cause of acne, and stimulants and sugar may be the reason.

Milk. There's something about milk that doesn't seem to apply to other dairy products in the causation of acne, and that may be lactose, a type of sugar, which is absent from fermented dairy products. Milk can cause acne whereas cheese, yogurt, butter, and cream don't seem to. Eliminate milk. Note that many people start the day with a bowl of sweetened cereal doused in milk, a perfect recipe for a spike in blood glucose and insulin and an acne breakout.

Industrial seed oils. Commonly known as vegetable oils, their high omega-6 content causes inflammation and metabolic syndrome which features acne-causing high insulin. Don't consume safflower, soy, corn, peanut, or canola oils. (Not an exhaustive list. Olive oil is acceptable.) Omega-3 fats (the kind in fish oil) may be protective.

Other, non-dietary, lifestyle factors can also affect acne.

Soap. Dermatologists recommend washing the face several times a day to eliminate oils and kill acne-causing bacteria. Bacteria don't live in a vacuum, however; they coexist with other bacteria in ecological balance. Soap upsets this balance by indiscriminately killing all bacteria, which may aggravate acne. I quit using soap on my face years ago, and that's worked very well for me. In fact, the combination of switching to a healthier diet and stopping the use of soap eliminated my adult acne. I wash my face with water only. If you have extremely oily skin, diet can help that a lot, but if it persists, washing with warm water may get rid of the remainder.

Sunshine. Getting out in the sun can clear acne, due to the bactericidal and anti-inflammatory effects of solar radiation. As with sun exposure in general, 10 or 15 minutes in the sun may be enough. Longer exposure risks burning, which should be avoided.

If you take care of all of the above dietary and lifestyle factors, but still have acne, some topical treatments can help. As with so many other supplements we've discussed in this book, the cheapest ones work best. Prescription anti-acne drugs such as Accutane have a raft of terrible side effects, including psychiatric effects – suicidal depression being one.[4] Long-term use of antibiotics for acne also leads to a host of problems.[5]

Benzoyl peroxide is the most common ingredient in over-the-counter acne treatments, as well as the cheapest, and it works. It's equally effective at concentrations of 2.5, 5.0, and 10%; since it can irritate skin, the lowest concentration may be best.[6] You don't need to spend 20 or 50 bucks or more to get effective acne treatment; most of those with benzoyl peroxide retail for a few dollars.

Salicylate is another common topical anti-acne treatment, is also cheap, and also works.[7]

The bacteria that cause acne need iron to grow and reproduce, as do all bacteria. Iron chelators, substances that bind and remove iron, greatly (4 to >20-fold) potentiate the effectiveness of topical anti-acne drugs like benzoyl peroxide.[8] (In fact, salicylate chelates iron.) Some topical acne treatments contain either green tea extract, tea tree oil, or other essential oils, and all of these fight acne at least in part by binding and removing iron. If you keep iron levels in the low normal range, as discussed in my book *Dumping Iron*, the skin also loses iron, and as a result, less acne could be a welcome side effect.

Acne – Key Points

- Diet strongly influences acne. Eliminate sugar, refined carbohydrates, seed oils, and milk to get rid of acne.

- Soap upsets the skin's microbial balance and may aggravate acne.
- Sunshine can treat acne.
- Inexpensive topical treatments that contain either benzoyl peroxide or salicylate are effective.

Acne is a disease of Western civilization; while there is a genetic component to acne, exposure to a Western lifestyle is also necessary. Change your lifestyle to eliminate acne.

Sun Damage and Wrinkles

Sun damage to skin is intimately connected to iron. Solar radiation, or any other kind of radiation, interacts with ferritin, which is the protein molecule that keeps highly reactive iron "locked down" and unavailable to react with other molecules. Radiation causes ferritin to release its iron, and free, highly reactive iron then causes skin damage. Free iron is a major factor, perhaps the most important one, in ultraviolet radiation damage to the skin.[9] Skin that's exposed to the sun has a higher iron content than skin that's not exposed.[10]

Substance that bind and remove iron (iron chelators) protect against sun damage.[11] One of the compounds that binds iron is kojic acid, a substance used in soap and cosmetic creams for skin lightening, most popularly in Japan.[12] Kojic acid appears to be effective at lightening the skin and removing iron; whether it would treat wrinkles or other damage that's already present does not seem to be known.

Niacinamide (also known as nicotinamide; no relation to nicotine) is a form of vitamin B3 that can effectively decrease skin wrinkles, in addition to treating blotches and hyperpigmented spots on skin.[13] A moisturizer that contained 4% niacinamide resulted in significant improvement in nearly 2/3 of the subjects tested. Topically applied IP6 (from rice bran, discussed in the chapter on supplements for long life) improves wrinkles too.[14] Lotions that contain resveratrol also protect the skin and may prevent photodamage; note that resveratrol is cheap, yet some retail products that contain it may cost hundreds of dollars, so look for a cheap one.

The substances that treat or protect against skin wrinkles and other damage are inexpensive; more expensive products offer little to no advantage over cheaper ones.

Baldness and Dandruff

Baldness seems to be a modern affliction that was much less common in the past, so modern lifestyle factors, especially dietary ones, could be responsible.

Male pattern baldness has been linked to an infection of the skin with the fungus *Malassezia furfur*; the antifungal drug ketoconazole kills this fungus and treats male pattern baldness just as well as the hair-growing drug minoxidil (Rogaine).[15]

"Comparative data suggest that there may be a significant action of KCZ [ketoconazole] upon the course of androgenic alopecia and that *Malassezia* spp. may play a role in the inflammatory reaction." (Quoting this so you know I'm not making it up, because most observers think that baldness is mysterious.)

If this holds true for many or all cases of male pattern baldness (androgenic alopecia), then our notions of why some men go bald (that it's due to testosterone metabolites) may be all wrong. Curiously, folklore has it that hats cause baldness — perhaps by giving fungus a warm, moist environment in which to grow?

If fungal infection in the skin causes both male pattern baldness and, as we'll see, dandruff, then iron is implicated, because all invasive microorganisms must acquire iron from their hosts. Male pattern baldness is also strongly linked to insulin resistance and metabolic syndrome.[16] The connection to insulin resistance provides a mechanism behind the fact that baldness is connected to a 2.5-fold greater risk of heart disease.[17]

Both dandruff and seborrheic dermatitis are linked to fungal infection by the fungus *Malassezia*.[18] All microorganisms that invade man and cause disease require iron. (Every living thing requires iron.) Withholding iron from microbes is at the center of an evolutionary arms race between mammals and bacteria and other microorganisms. Donating blood could treat fungal infections of the skin by lowering skin iron levels, and maybe baldness too, although both of those are conjecture. (Nevertheless, a reader of my website told me that his seborrheic dermatitis of many years standing, which nothing would treat, disappeared after he started donating blood.)

Shampoo that contains salicylate and ciclopirox effectively treats dandruff.[19] Ciclopirox is an iron chelator (it attaches to and removes iron), as is salicylate. By attaching and removing iron, they deprive fungus of required growth material, it dies, and dandruff goes away. Ketoconazole, an anti-fungal chemical that works by inhibiting fungal steroid synthesis, also treats dandruff.

Topical agents that either kill fungi, remove iron from the skin, or both, may treat not only dandruff, but may be useful against baldness as well.

Essential oils, such as rosemary, sage, oregano, and coriander may also treat baldness (as they do for acne). A trial of rosemary oil versus minoxidil in male pattern baldness resulted in both groups having significant hair growth in 6 months, and there was no difference between groups, although the minoxidil group reported greater itching.[20] So, rosemary oil may be even better than minoxidil. The essential oils laurel, sage, rosemary, oregano, and coriander all kill fungi, with oregano oil being the most potent.[21] That suggests that they could all be active against male pattern baldness. (Another reader of my website grew back his hair by using rosemary oil.)

To summarize, both male pattern baldness and dandruff are linked to fungal infection and iron. Genetic factors are important too, as the fungus *Malassezia* is a common one that can colonize the skin of healthy people. Essential oils such as rosemary oil, and shampoos that contain anti-fungal ingredients, may treat both conditions.

Which brings us to shampoo. I don't use it, and neither do lots of other people.

The scalp produces oils that then coat the hair, and other things being equal, there seems no reason to periodically – for most people daily – remove that oil with shampoo, as well as to effectively sterilize the scalp. The health of the scalp and hair requires the oil and microorganisms. Omitting shampoo, or using it less often, means you aren't exposed to as many synthetic chemicals either, some of which are endocrine disruptors that have estrogen activity and could lead to disruption of male hormones.

Try washing your hair in water only, or, if you have very oily hair and scalp, wash less often. If you do use shampoo, find one without the harmful chemicals. For most men, using shampoo less often or not at all will present no difficulties because they typically wear their hair short.

And to extend the comparison, the same applies to soap as well. Stepping into a hot shower and soaping up your body kills the microbes on the skin, which are normally there for a reason and are important in keeping skin healthy. If you wouldn't take antibiotics daily to "clean" your gut, another body site that's normally full of microbes, why would you want to sterilize your skin daily? As I wrote above, stopping the use of soap on my face cleared up my acne, probably by restoring a healthy microbial balance; soon after I took the hint and stopped using soap on the rest of my body.

Grey Hair

Grey hair is obviously associated with aging. In aging, there's an increase in oxidative stress, which means the inability of cells in the body to properly control excess oxygen radicals. It makes sense that this is involved in grey hair, since both bleach and hydrogen peroxide cause a loss of color by generating oxygen.

A few years ago, scientists got to the root of the gray hair problem: hydrogen peroxide in the scalp causes greying hair. In essence, higher levels of oxidative stress in the hair shaft cause a loss of the activities of antioxidant enzymes, resulting in the accumulation of hydrogen peroxide and the loss of melanocyte (cells that produce color) activity. However, other researchers in this area point to multiple causes of gray hair. Another recent report confirmed that oxidative stress lies behind gray hair, and this is due to far lower levels of antioxidant activity in the hair follicle. Involvement of copper and thyroid hormones has also been fingered.

The big question that remains is whether damage done to hair follicles can be reversed. If melanocytes are destroyed, then the damage probably cannot be reversed, since this would involve growing new melanocytes, presumably from stem cells.

If the melanocytes are merely overwhelmed by hydrogen peroxide and temporarily out of commission, then reversal may be possible. I doubt if anyone has the answer to that one. Would it be possible to boost antioxidant activity in the hair follicle? Maybe. It's definitely possible to boost overall antioxidant activity, but whether this would affect the hair follicle is unknown. Perhaps something would need to be applied topically, something that can be absorbed through the skin.

Grey hair is so closely associated with the physiological processes of aging that anything that fights aging ought to affect greying. But again, whether grey hair is the result of permanent damage or can be cured is unknown at this point.

I'm already doing just about everything I can in the way of health, and I noticed my hair darkening somewhat after I got my iron levels lower, but most of the grey still persists. I'm not holding my breath for dark hair, and I don't think it's that big of a deal anyway. Better to work on more important things that you have some control over, like body composition, health, learning, and charisma.

Skin and Hair – Key Points

- A poor diet with sugar and vegetable oils promotes acne
- Getting sunshine and omitting soap can help treat acne
- Benzoyl peroxide and salicylate are the cheapest and most effective anti-acne meds
- Niacinamide and kojic acid may treat wrinkled skin
- Male pattern baldness and dandruff may both be caused by iron excess and fungal infection
- Essential oils can promote hair growth
- Soap – do you really need it?
- Grey hair: we haven't figured that one out yet so you're on your own.

8: Alcohol

Alcohol, while not a supplement, is a widely-used drug. Many studies have shown that alcohol is associated with better health and longer life, yet because epidemiological studies can't show causation, and because many confounding factors that differ between drinkers and non-drinkers could skew results, the effects of alcohol on health remain subject to a great deal of uncertainty. Many people, having read media accounts of the benefits of alcohol, just assume that drinking is healthy, but in reality, the case for alcohol isn't quite so simple. In this chapter, I'll discuss the effects of alcohol, both good and bad, and try to sort out whether alcohol truly benefits health.

Researchers have long known that moderate drinkers tend to live longer than either non-drinkers or heavy drinkers, and by now, countless studies have been done on the relation of alcohol with health. Moderate drinkers are particularly less likely to have coronary heart disease, and since this is the number one killer in the U.S. today, reductions in heart disease mean that drinkers would be likely to live longer, even if alcohol caused other health problems.

A meta-analysis (a study of other studies) found that the lowest risk of heart disease was in drinkers of up to 20 grams of alcohol daily, and their risk was 20% lower than non-drinkers. (One "standard drink" contains 14 grams of alcohol, hence 20 grams is less than two drinks.) Yet there was still a protective effect, that is, a lower risk of heart disease than non-drinkers, at amounts of up to 72 grams daily, or about 5 drinks.[1] Binge drinking, on the other hand, is associated with much worse health, as you might expect.

The relation between alcohol consumption and total mortality, that is, death from any cause, not merely heart disease, was studied by a large meta-analysis published in the Archives of Internal Medicine.[2] It concluded that there was a J-shaped relation between death rates and alcohol consumption: as consumption increased from zero, risk of death dropped, but then as consumption increased further, risk rose again. The maximum decrease in the death rate was 18% for women and 17% for men; up to 4 drinks a day for men, and 2 for women, offered some degree of protection.

Studies like these have not only found fairly large reductions in death rates from drinking alcohol, but they've also found that even a high number of daily drinks, up to 4 or even 5, means protection against death. (I don't know about you, but I consider 4 or 5 daily drinks a high number.) Mainstream media reports, as well as pronouncements from on high by various doctors and organizations, would lead you to believe that only 1 or 2 daily drinks (in men) is the most you can drink for health benefits, i.e. "light" or "moderate" drinking. But going by a strict interpretation of the evidence, they may be underplaying the benefits of alcohol. While 1 to 2 drinks may confer maximum benefits compared to zero or more than 2 drinks, drinking up to 4 to 5 drinks a day still correlates with better health than drinking no alcohol.

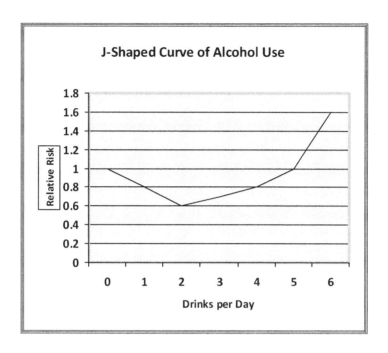

Health organizations and doctors have been rather subdued in commenting on the benefits of moderate drinking because a) they don't want to make statements that go beyond the evidence, and as we'll see, the evidence contains more than meets the eye; and b) they don't want to encourage drinking for fear of promoting addictive behaviors and alcoholism. These are laudable goals, no doubt, even if there's a bit of subterfuge embedded in them.

Why studies on alcohol can't necessarily be taken at face value

Epidemiology studies, like those finding that moderate drinkers have better health than non-drinkers, can't prove that alcohol *causes* the benefits to health. They only show an association, drinking on the one hand, better health on the other. There could be a number of reasons why alcohol does *not* cause better health; other characteristics of both drinkers and non-drinkers may account for the results.

Non-drinkers could be of two kinds: either they have never drunk alcohol in their lives, or they quit drinking at some point. People who have quit drinking are likely to have done so because of health problems or alcoholism; so here's a case where non-drinkers may have worse health and skew the results toward worse health being associated with no drinking, but it's not abstention from alcohol that causes poor health; they either had poor health to begin with or alcohol caused it.

Even lifelong non-drinkers (teetotalers) may have worse health than drinkers not because they abstain, but because they have inborn characteristics that, in part, make them more likely to abstain, and lead to worse health. Intelligence (IQ) and socioeconomic status are the most important characteristics that differ between drinkers and non-drinkers, and they can both skew results highly. Contrary to common belief, more intelligent and wealthier people drink more than those with a lower IQ and lower income, not less.[3] In turn, intelligence and socioeconomic status predict health.[4] People with higher intelligence may take better care of themselves, or they may have been born with better health, their higher intelligence merely being an indication of a well-functioning brain, and the body is therefore working better and is less prone to disease.

Yet another confounding factor concerns the type of alcohol consumed. For example, a Danish study found that drinking from 3 to 5 glasses of red wine daily was associated with about half the death rate compared to no drinking, while beer had no effect, and drinking a similar quantity of spirits *increased* the risk of death.[5] Red wine contains grape polyphenols that are associated with better health, and beer and spirits do not. There's even another confounding factor built in here, and that is that more intelligent and wealthier people are more likely to drink red wine rather than other types of alcoholic drinks.

The Mediterranean diet may offer protection against heart disease and cancer; at least, people who eat in that style have less disease and better health. High adherence to a Mediterranean diet is associated with a 15% lower death rate.[6] One of the main features of a Mediterranean diet is the consumption of red wine; in fact, alcohol consumption accounted for 23.5% of its effects, making it the most important component of the diet.

Red wine contains polyphenols from grapes that promote vascular health and may help prevent cancer. While alcohol itself upregulates stress defense via hormesis, red wine polyphenols alone can inhibit atherosclerosis, as shown by the fact that non-alcoholic red wine (and grape juice) can do this.[7]

Alcohol use is associated with higher cancer rates. "[D]rinking on average 25 grams of pure alcohol per day [less than 2 drinks] was associated with significantly elevated cancer risks for the following sites: oral cavity and pharynx, esophagus, stomach, colon and rectum, liver, larynx, and female breast. [ref. 1]"

That's a lot of confounding.

And yet, in male twins who were discordant in alcohol use – that is, one abstained, the other drank – the abstaining twin was twice as likely to die first, which indicates that genetics may not entirely explain differences in health with alcohol use.[8] Furthermore, even lifelong non-drinkers, i.e. not ex-drinkers who may have quit for health reasons, had worse health than moderate drinkers.[9]

Can we make any sense out of the relation between alcohol and health? Unfortunately, the issue is not settled, but we can make some informed speculation.

In testing in lab animals, alcohol improves health markers, and the non-alcoholic components of red wine do that as well. Alcohol also inhibits mTOR, the biochemical mechanism strongly implicated in aging, and that could well account for much of its health benefit.[10] So there are good reasons to think that alcohol has health benefits; if alcohol did not protect health as measured in the laboratory, and worsened measures of health, then we would be right to be skeptical of the epidemiology research. But that is not the case.

While confounding in those epidemiology studies undoubtedly exists, studies in twins and in groups similar in intelligence and socioeconomic factors (e.g. male British doctors[11]), which limit confounding factors such as genetics, IQ, and socioeconomic status, show a protective effect of alcohol.

I conclude that alcohol protects health and lowers death rates, but possibly not quite to the extent found in some of the studies, and red wine is more protective than other forms of alcohol.

How much alcohol is too much?

When drunk to excess and over a long period of time, alcohol can damage the liver, as well as increase cancer risk. Whether alcohol causes better health or whether it merely associates with it, we do know that heavy drinking causes disease. But what constitutes heavy drinking?

Perhaps the most serious disease associated with alcohol is cirrhosis of the liver, in which the liver becomes scarred and fibrotic and loses function. One consequence of cirrhosis is bleeding, since the liver makes blood clotting factors.

Hard-core alcoholics sometimes require blood transfusions. I once asked a doctor friend who sometimes treated these people how much drinking was necessary to cause the need for a transfusion.

His reply: a bottle of liquor a day for ten years.

That's a lot of booze. My own research into this issue has led me to believe that the doctor's estimate is indeed in the ballpark.

A German doctor studied hundreds of alcoholics at a clinic over the course of many years, and published his results.[12] Several factors must be taken into account for the study of alcohol and its relation to health and disease. Among these are

- amount
- lifetime duration
- intensity

Getting a handle on these is difficult due to high variation among drinkers, recalling amounts and times, differences in the type of alcohol, male vs female, etc.

The doctor charted the incidence of liver cirrhosis against lifetime alcohol intake, and helpfully translated it into lifetime equivalent intake of liters of 100 proof whiskey.

At a total lifetime intake of 7,100 liters of 100 proof whiskey, you're practically guaranteed to get cirrhosis. However, 50% of the alcoholics had cirrhosis at an intake of about 2,000 liters.

That's a lot of drinking.

Nevertheless, it's estimated that only between 8 and 30% of alcoholics show signs of liver damage. Some drinkers got liver damage at much lower levels of drinking. What accounts for this?

One variant between people who experience liver damage and those who don't may be diet. Dietary saturated fat protects rats from alcohol-induced liver disease. In fact, saturated fats not only protect, but reverse it.[13] Rats fed both ethanol continuously plus palm oil showed a reversal in liver damage due to down-regulation of COX-2 and TNF alpha. Rats that were fed ethanol plus fish oil showed the worst liver damage. In another experiment by the same group, beef tallow wholly prevented alcoholic liver disease in rats, whereas those fed corn oil got a severe case of it.[14]

So, it could be that among humans, those who get cirrhosis eat a high amount of polyunsaturated fats and junk food. Those who don't may eat lots of meat and butter.

We now have a ballpark figure of how much alcohol causes severe liver damage. Generally, it's a lot, but there's also a wide variation.

What about "normal" drinking, say, a couple glasses of wine or a couple cocktails in the evening — does that have a potential to cause damage?

A "standard drink" in the U.S. is deemed to contain 14 grams of pure ethanol. Translated into everyday terms, a standard drink is

- one 12-ounce beer, if that beer is 5% alcohol
- one glass (5 ounces) of wine, at 12% alcohol
- 1.5 ounces of spirits, at 40% alcohol

In "A meta-analysis of alcohol consumption and the risk of 15 diseases"[15], the authors found "strong trends in risk... for cancers of the oral cavity, esophagus and larynx, hypertension, liver cirrhosis, chronic pancreatitis, and injuries and violence. Less strong direct relations were observed for cancers of the colon, rectum, liver, and breast. For all these conditions, significant increased risks were also found for ethanol intake of 25 g per day."

Significantly increased risks were found at consumption of more than 25 grams of ethanol daily, that is, the amount in about 2 drinks. They found a protective effect of alcohol only for coronary heart disease, with a minimum risk at up to 20 grams of ethanol daily, or less than 2 drinks — although up to 72 grams a day, or about 5 drinks, still showed protection against heart disease.

While heart disease is the leading killer of Americans, cancer isn't far behind.

If you're in shape, eat right, exercise regularly, do the important things for your health, you're likely at low risk for heart disease already. Drinking alcohol won't offer you additional protection from heart disease. It will, however, increase your risk of cancer and a number of other diseases.

Regular drinking also has a significant effect in raising blood pressure. However, blood pressure drops rapidly upon cessation of or even cutting back on drinking, within a few days.[16] Alcohol consumption increased blood pressure only if that consumption was in the 3 days prior to blood pressure testing. If the consumption was prior to 3 days before examination, no effect was seen. If you've been told you have high blood pressure, and you drink alcohol, abstaining from drinking for a few days and retesting may be wise. It could save you from being medicated for it with drugs that have a high incidence of adverse side effects, like fatigue.

From all of the above, you can see that alcohol is a mixed bag, decreasing the rate of some diseases, mainly heart disease, and raising the risks of others, such as cancer. The decision whether to drink alcohol is highly individual, one that no one else can make. While alcohol may not be as healthy as some would have you believe, one can take some consolation that it may not be as unhealthy as others want you to believe.

From all the evidence, red wine appears to be the healthiest drink, with health benefits from grape polyphenols in addition to alcohol. Spirits are the unhealthiest; beer is neutral – although beer may cause the most weight gain, due to a high content of maltose, a sugar. Cocktails made with sweet mixes, such as a margarita or a gin and tonic, arguably fall into last place on the health scale.

If you do drink alcohol, a couple glasses of red wine appear to offer the greatest benefit with the least risk.

Alcohol and weight gain

Scientists recently showed that a so-called fasting-mimicking diet had beneficial effects on various biomarkers of aging in both mice and humans; this diet was low calorie, low protein, and designed to induce ketosis and reduce growth hormone axis signaling.

Alcohol is low protein, low carb, and low fat; in fact, pure alcohol contains zero of these macronutrients. Maybe consuming calories from alcohol counts toward a fasting-mimicking diet and helps reverse aging.

There are three basic macronutrients from which higher organisms get sustenance; carbohydrate, protein, and fat. A fourth is alcohol. Some say that alcohol is not a macronutrient, since we don't need it to survive, but we don't need dietary carbohydrate to survive, so then that wouldn't be a macronutrient either.

Alcohol metabolizes into acetaldehyde, a relatively toxic product, and the acetaldehyde is in turn made into acetate, from which energy can be derived. However, the acetate appears mainly to be just burned as energy rather than stored; the acetate could also feed into a metabolic pathway that makes fat.

A number of studies have found that alcohol intake is not associated with weight gain.[17] The reasons appear to be two: drinkers compensate for alcoholic calorie consumption by eating less, and alcoholic calories appear to inefficiently metabolized. As I wrote above, these calories may be stored as fat only with difficulty, which agrees with the idea of inefficient metabolism. The report states, "Ethanol is not stored in the body, but it is oxidized in preference over other fuels." Some studies have found, however, that heavy drinkers (more than 3 drinks a day) do tend to have a higher body weight.

Alcoholic drinks, as opposed to pure ethanol, vary widely in the number of calories, sugar, and other nutrient sources. For instance, a White Russian has 257 calories, much of it from sugar. This probably explains Lebowski's weight problem. A hot buttered rum comes in at 316. A beer comes in at 155 calories, but beer contains maltose, a sugar, which promotes weight gain.

By contrast, hard liquor contains calories only from ethanol. A scotch contains 80 calories, and this would be roughly the same for a shot of vodka, gin, or rum.

Red wine is similar; a 5-ounce glass contains 85 calories.

So, weight gain could vary tremendously depending on what one's drink of choice is.

The lesson here is, I believe, that if you drink and want to stay lean, choose plain highballs, such as a scotch on the rocks or something similar, or dry red wine. Avoid drinks with added sugar, such as margaritas, gin and tonics, or White Russians. Beer is probably best avoided too. Sugar in mixed drinks, not ethanol, most likely causes weight gain. If you want to stay lean and muscular, choose plain highballs or dry red wine if you drink.

Alcohol – Key Points

- Alcohol research is confounded by many factors
- Different types of alcohol may have different effects
- Evidence points to red wine as the healthiest
- 2 drinks a day are associated with greatest reduction in health risks
- Binge and excessive drinking is still bad for you – sorry
- Alcohol may not cause weight gain, depending on choice of tipple

9: Supplements to Avoid

We've discussed the benefits of many supplements, but there are a number of supplements that have little benefit or may even be harmful; some of them shouldn't be used unless you've got good reason, others that you should avoid entirely. The problem with bad supplements partly stems from mainstream ideas of what's good for you (e.g. calcium), others come from hucksters eager to make a buck off the public's ignorance (e.g. sports drinks and pre-workout supplements). Some of them you should avoid because they provide no benefit, and are thus a waste of money; others may be actually harmful to health.

Calcium

Calcium is a mineral (a metal) that is important in bone function and strength, and in other important physiological processes. It's widely prescribed, and many people, especially women, take it on their own for its alleged effect on osteoporosis, which is the thinning of bones with age.

Unfortunately, calcium supplements don't improve osteoporosis. A meta-analysis of studies on calcium intake and risk of hip or other bone fracture concluded that there was no benefit and possibly even increased risk:

Pooled results from randomized controlled trials show no reduction in hip fracture risk with calcium supplementation, and an increased risk is possible. For any nonvertebral fractures, there was a neutral effect in the randomized trials.[1]

Why would there be no benefit at best? One reason may be that lack of calcium doesn't cause osteoporosis or hip fractures; lack of weight-bearing exercise, dietary protein, and vitamins D and K may be much more important. Just throwing some calcium into the body doesn't help bones; unless a real calcium deficiency exists, more calcium doesn't build stronger bones.

On the other hand, calcium supplements may increase risk of other health problems. Calcium is implicated in coronary artery disease; calcification of arteries features in this disease.

Calcium builds up in the lining of arteries, making them stiff and bone-like. Calcium in the coronary arteries strongly predicts cardiovascular events such as heart attacks, and in those without other known risk factors, it is in fact the strongest predictor.[2] The test called CAC measures this, the initials standing for coronary artery calcium.

Calcium supplementation is associated with an increased risk of heart attack: a meta-analysis found that people allocated to a calcium supplement had about a 30% increased risk of heart attack compared to placebo:[3]

*As calcium supplements are widely used these modest increases in risk of cardiovascular disease might translate into a large burden of disease in the population. **A reassessment of the role of calcium supplements in the management of osteoporosis is warranted.***

Another study found more than double the risk of heart attack in users of calcium supplements.[4]

Calcium can increase the risk of other diseases as well, leading to an increased death rate. Use of calcium supplements along with dietary calcium intake of greater than 1400 mg a day was associated with a 2.5-fold increased risk of death.[5]

Unless you have a very good reason, such as a doctor's orders, avoid calcium supplements. If your doctor wants you to take them, be sure you understand why.

An irony regarding calcium supplementation is that increased consumption of dairy products, which contain lots of calcium, is associated with much lower death rates.[6] The reason that dairy is protective may have nothing to do with calcium, but with other components of dairy, such as protein and fat, or vitamin K.[7] Dairy products also inhibit iron absorption, which may have a lot to do with their health benefits.

Clearly, the problem isn't normally whether someone is getting enough calcium, but ensuring that the calcium goes to the right places: bones and not arteries. Vitamin K helps to ensure that calcium goes where it belongs, and higher intake is associated with greater bone mineral density. Vitamin D is also much more helpful for bone density than calcium.

The tragedy here is that doctors routinely prescribe calcium supplements to older people, especially women, who are at greater risk of osteoporosis, another reason why you have to educate yourself. Many people also blindly pop calcium supplements in response to decades of bad advice that calcium is good for them. Don't be one of them. In reality, not many people who eat good diets suffer from a calcium deficiency.

Be aware that virtually all multi-vitamins contain a hefty dose of calcium, although usually not as much as in an actual calcium supplement tablet.

Iron

I've written about iron extensively, an entire book in fact.[8] Getting and maintaining iron levels in the low normal range may make the difference in whether you are free of disease and healthy, or not. That's especially important for men, who have higher iron levels than women, on average.

Some knowledgeable observers of iron and health, such as Dr. Eugene Weinberg, who's spent his academic career studying the relation between excess iron and disease, believe that much of the problem of iron overload in the American population is driven by iron supplements, rather than diet.[9] The body maintains iron absorption within a range, but excess iron from supplements or iron-fortified food may override this mechanism. Most multivitamins contain iron, and doctors widely prescribe iron to women, even when they're post-menopausal and rarely need it. Doctors also prescribe them to older people for anemia, even when the anemia's cause is unlikely to be iron deficiency.

Iron overload is dangerous and begins at a level much lower than most doctors believe. To measure iron, doctors and laboratories normally measure ferritin, the protein that stores iron within the body. The laboratory normal ranges for ferritin have far too high an upper limit consistent with good health. I won't rehash all the reasons that excess iron is bad for health – though I'll urge you to read my book on that subject – but suffice to say here that excess iron is associated with heart disease, cancer, diabetes, infections, and many other nasty conditions.

So don't take iron supplements unless you have a demonstrated need and a doctor prescribes them to you. Demonstrated need usually means iron-deficiency anemia, which is characterized by low hemoglobin and microcytic red blood cells. Be sure you understand exactly why they're being prescribed.

Many people take iron supplements on their own, however, which isn't a good idea, and harmful to health in most cases. Many also take it without knowing, because most multivitamins contain iron. For men over 20 years of age and women over 50 who want to take a multivitamin, a "mature" multivitamin is a better bet, since these normally don't contain iron. (Most of them also contain calcium, however, which as we noted above, isn't a good idea either.)

Beware of iron-fortified foods, the equivalent to taking an iron supplement. Some breakfast cereals contain 100% of the daily requirement of iron, which is in addition to being made with iron-fortified flour or corn meal to begin with. (Anyway, breakfast cereal isn't even real food, it will spike your blood glucose and insulin and make you fat.) The U.S. government mandates by law that all flour, corn meal, and rice be fortified with iron.

In the days when people were poor, couldn't afford to eat much meat, and had intestinal parasites, iron deficiency was a much bigger problem. It's less of a problem now, the condition mainly being confined to a small percentage of women of child-bearing age. In the U.S., Europe, and other places in the developed world, it's difficult to get an inadequate amount of dietary iron. The problem now is the reverse, too much iron.

Copper

Copper is a somewhat overlooked but required mineral. Not too many people knowingly take copper supplements, but multivitamins often contain it.

High levels of copper are associated with large increases in death from cancer, more than double the rate of people with low levels.[10] Copper is also associated with increased risk of Alzheimer's disease, atherosclerosis, and diabetes.[11] It can induce premature senescence in cells.[12]

People with the highest levels of copper probably got to that level by taking copper supplements, either directly or inadvertently. Old copper pipes can also add a significant amount of copper to drinking water.

Copper, like iron, is a reactive metal, so it's not surprising that high levels will increase health risks. One of the few times that copper supplements may be needed is with high doses of zinc, since zinc blocks copper absorption. In fact, high-dose zinc is used as a treatment for Wilson's disease, which is characterized by an overload of copper. Sometimes it's said that if you supplement with high-dose zinc, you should take a copper supplement too so you can avoid zinc toxicity, but a better idea would be to avoid high-dose zinc supplementation.

Watch for copper in multivitamins. Again, mature multivitamins – some of them anyway – may be formulated without copper.

Metal Overload

Calcium, iron, and copper supplements are associated with health risks and you should avoid them except under a doctor's orders.

Is it a coincidence that all three of these are metals? I don't think it is. Iron as a driver of aging may possibly be generalized to **a metal overload theory** – although we need these metals and can become deficient in them, too much of them is a bad thing.

We need these metals abundantly as we're growing, to provide materials for bones and blood and muscles. After we stop growing, these metals accumulate in our bodies and accelerate aging. There's a good case to be made that they actually cause aging.

While too much of anything can harm us, we seem to be particularly susceptible to metal overload, since we have no regulated way of eliminating them from our bodies. They build up as we age, and the excess causes damage to health.

Antioxidants

Really? You're going to tell me not to take antioxidants, which every media outlet constantly touts as healthy, and have said so for decades?

Really.

Not only are antioxidants unnecessary, but they may even increase death rates, and they probably hinder the health benefits of exercise.

Antioxidants are natural or chemical substances that quench free radicals and therefore, in theory, prevent damage to cells, improve health, and fight aging. The most well-known antioxidants are vitamins C and E. While these two are required nutrients, they have a downside when taken in excessive amounts.

Free radicals, or more technically, reactive oxygen species, are molecules created inside cells as a result of metabolism, and that can cause damage.

Free radicals were long thought to be a primary driver of aging; the theory is no longer widely held, since free radicals act as signaling molecules in cells, as it's been discovered, and are necessary for health. While free radicals can damage cells, other processes are more important to aging, although exactly which ones are most important is the subject of intense debate among scientists.

Exercise and other forms of stress generate free radicals that then cause hormesis, which is the upgrading of cellular defense mechanisms caused by a stress or toxin. Hormesis, whether through exercise or other means, strengthens the organism by making it more stress resistant and able to withstand bigger stresses down the road. Stress resistance combats aging, and loss of it is highly implicated in aging.

Blunting or abolishing the free radicals produced by exercise means blunting or abolishing most or all of the healthful effects of exercise. Exercise depends at least in part on the generation of free radicals to improve health. Vitamins C and E, when taken regularly and/or around exercise, can completely negate the health benefits of exercise.[13] Research on this topic is ongoing, and some researchers have not found this effect; nevertheless, as we'll see below, there are good reasons to believe that it occurs.

No exercise-induced hormesis means little or no improvement in health from exercise. The body *must* sense exercise as stressful in order for it to increase exercise capacity, mitochondrial function, and lifespan.

It doesn't take large amounts of vitamins C and E to hamper the effects of exercise either; 1000 mg of vitamin C and 235 mg of vitamin E will prevent the increase in mitochondria that exercise normally promotes.

Many athletes and others who exercise a lot often take these vitamins, and that doesn't seem like a great idea. They may be hampering their training profoundly, although there might be the upside of preventing colds or other upper respiratory tract infections, which hard-training athletes often get.

Furthermore, and perhaps even more alarming, a meta-analysis of antioxidant trials found that taking antioxidant supplements was associated with an *increased* risk of death.[14] Vitamin C and selenium had no association with increased or decreased risk, but vitamin A was associated with a 16% increased risk of death, vitamin E with a 4% increased risk, and beta carotene with 7% increased risk.

What's going on here? Evidently, free radicals are so necessary for health that quenching may result in worse health and higher risk of death. The zero effect of vitamin C and selenium in decreasing risk might mean that, if not actively harmful, they don't do much good either.

Antioxidants inhibit autophagy

Antioxidants also inhibit autophagy and this effect, along with the blunting of the healthful effects of exercise, could be behind the increased risk of death found in the meta-analysis.[15]

Autophagy is the cellular self-cleansing process that rids cells of junk, and thus repairs damage, and is extremely important in the aging process. The rate of autophagy declines with age, and keeping the rate at high levels is critical for slowing aging, and can be done with intermittent fasting, a low-carbohydrate diet, and/or autophagy boosters.

The study cited above found that the efficacy of drugs that induce autophagy, including rapamycin and trehalose, can be impaired by antioxidants.

The ability of fasting to induce autophagy is also impaired by antioxidants.

Does this mean you should never take antioxidants? No, it doesn't, but caution is in order.

Vitamin C

Up to 22% of apparently healthy people in the United States are deficient in vitamin C, and provision of vitamin C at 1,000 mg daily to those who are deficient increases the level of physical activity and reduces the incidence and duration of the common cold by almost 50%.[16] Those are not small effects, and if you suffer from frequent colds or fatigue, vitamin C may be worth taking. Taking 6 to 8 grams of vitamin C daily at the onset of a cold can reduce its duration by 20%.[17]

In hospitalized patients, 500 mg of vitamin C, twice a day, improved mood.[18]

Most impressive of all is the effect of vitamin C in sepsis, a serious and often fatal illness in which bacteria or other microorganisms infect the blood stream. When doctors administered 6 grams of vitamin C intravenously, 4 times a day, along with thiamine and hydrocortisone, the number of deaths in septic patients dropped by nearly 90%.[19] Giving vitamin C intravenously is the only way to get blood levels of the vitamin high, so this isn't something you'd try at home. But it's worth noting here in case you or a loved one are in this situation, and suggest that the doctor do this. Most will not do so on their own, although the dramatic results of this study suggest that this vitamin C treatment could become more widespread and accepted.

If you are in otherwise good health and have enough vitamin C, extra amounts may do little and may decrease the health benefits of your exercise.

Muscle contains a large amount of vitamin C, so here's another area where supplementing a deficient person could help, but it's unlikely to make a difference in muscle to those who have a sufficient amount.

The only way to tell if you're vitamin C deficient is through a lab test. Taking small doses, 500 mg or under, may be a good trial to see if it improves your health or mood.

Another of the antioxidants that inhibited autophagy was n-acetylcysteine (NAC). This cysteine pro-drug replenishes glutathione, the body's most abundant internal antioxidant, which is necessary for good health. While NAC can be useful in the treatment of mental and physical disorders, having too much glutathione may be as detrimental as too little. Caution is in order if taking NAC as well.

If you want to take vitamins C and E for any reason, don't take them immediately before or after exercise, and do not take them while fasting. They should be taken, if needed, during the fed state, i.e. during or within a few hours after a meal.

Dose is another consideration. If you have the symptoms of vitamin C deficiency and want to supplement with it, smaller doses, say a couple hundred milligrams daily, may be better. Don't use large doses unless you have good reason, such as a serious illness or infection.

Antioxidants are misnamed

The notion of antioxidants as healthful is so ingrained, and the idea that healthful effects of various foods are due to antioxidants so established, that we often hear that something is good for us due to high levels of antioxidants.

That is not the case.

Plant foods such as blueberries, broccoli, red wine, chocolate, and coffee have health benefits not because of antioxidant content, which is low, but because they contain phytochemicals that upgrade stress defense mechanisms. It used to be thought that quenching of free radicals lay behind the health effects of phytochemicals, but that no longer seems tenable. In effect, these foods, blueberries, broccoli, etc., contain low-dose toxins.

So, next time you read, e.g. "coffee is the biggest source of antioxidants for Americans", or "eat these high-antioxidant blueberries", understand that these statements are misleading.

They contain low levels of antioxidants, but contain high levels of phytochemicals that promote hormesis. By all means include them in your diet, because they promote health, but they don't do so because of antioxidants.

Antioxidants are not nearly as health-promoting as we've been led to believe, and may in some cases be harmful to health.

Designer Steroids, Peptides, Growth Hormone Promoters, and SARMs

There are many types of anabolic steroids, which are drugs that mimic and/or exaggerate the muscle-building and masculinizing effects of testosterone. Since most known steroids have been banned from sports, some athletes seek out ways to boost their performance with unbanned, or undetectable steroids.

Furthermore, not all steroids have been made illegal. New types of steroids pop up, and lawmakers might not get around to making them illegal for a while.

This is the world of designer steroids, where chemists synthesize molecules that have anabolic effects but which are either not detectable via standard laboratory analysis or which are legal, at least for the time being.

Some of these designer steroids may even work well, others may not. But you really don't know what you're getting. And even if they do work, they're still steroids, which carry health risks, and are definitely not anti-aging drugs. Pro-aging is more like it.

So, you may see various places online selling "muscle-building" "supplements", but they're really drugs, may be effective or not, and may damage your health. Use of designer steroids seems like a really bad idea.

Another, similar category is that of peptides, which are small protein molecules that promote endogenous hormone production, for example, of growth hormone. Since peptides do not survive digestion intact, they must be injected. Other, non-peptide substances, such as ibutamoren or MK-677, also promote the body's own growth hormone production; non-peptide substances normally do not require injection.

While promotion of endogenous growth hormone production could have important medical uses, such as in growth hormone deficient people, exogenous growth hormone in normally healthy people promotes aging and disease. Whether extra growth hormone produced by the body itself has that effect is not known with certainty, but seems likely. Longer life is associated with *less* growth hormone, within certain limits, i.e. a very low level may not be healthy either. Unless and until much more is known about increasing the body's own growth hormone production via drugs, it would be wise to avoid these growth hormone promoters.

Selective androgen receptor modulators, or SARMs, have some of the effects of steroids but not others. They depend on the different types of androgen (testosterone) receptors in different tissues; for example, muscle androgen receptors differ from androgen receptors in the prostate gland. SARMs bind to androgen receptors in muscle and promote muscle growth, while potentially having few if any other effects on other tissues, effects such as virilization or behavioral changes. As noted above, anabolic steroids also have androgenic effects; SARMs, in theory, have only anabolic effects, and little to no androgenic effects.

SARMs hold promise for muscle growth in both the elderly and infirm, and in cancer patients who suffer cachexia. In both of these groups, loss of muscle and other lean tissue compromises quality of life, and in cancer patients may even hasten death. Sarcopenia, or muscle wasting, is common in the elderly; in cancer, preservation of muscle may mean better ability to withstand treatment. Preservation and growth of lean mass in these groups is desirable, and a SARM, ostarine (also known as enobosarm), has been shown to increase muscle mass in healthy elderly people.[20] The benefits were modest, with men at the highest dose gaining 1.4 kg (3.1 pounds) lean mass in 3 months and losing about 0.3 kg of fat, and without any strength training. Ostarine was well-tolerated, but one subject had to discontinue the drug due to elevated liver enzymes (indicating liver injury); his enzymes returned to normal after cessation of the drug. Insulin resistance and triglycerides both decreased, and these are beneficial effects, to be expected with more muscle and less fat mass.

Various outlets now sell ostarine, with the idea that it will help bodybuilders or other strength athletes build muscle. Unfortunately for that idea, it's not known whether ostarine will do that in men who are already maximizing muscle mass via lifting weights and adequate protein intake. In people who have a pathologically low amount of muscle mass, ostarine works; but would those people have low lean mass had they been lifting weights and eating enough protein? (Not everyone is healthy enough to undertake strength training, of course.) Resistance (strength) training for 3 months in someone new to the activity, along with adequate protein and calorie intake, would likely add just as much or more lean mass as ostarine did in the same time frame. Would ostarine add muscle in veteran strength athletes? Maybe, but in my opinion that's doubtful, and in any case, we don't know, unless and until it's tested clinically on athletes. And that will probably never happen.

Furthermore, ostarine has only been tested in one small clinical trial for a short term; we don't know what long-term effects of this drug might be. It's possible that, like steroids or exogenous growth hormone, it might turn out to have unwanted and deleterious side effects. The highest dose used in the trial was 3 mg, yet some bodybuilders advocate taking as much as 75 mg a day.

Ostarine has not been shown more effective than lifting weights and adequate protein intake; the case for the use of ostarine to enhance muscle growth in bodybuilders and strength trainers has not been shown either; and we don't know what the long-term effects, or the effects of high doses, are. Therefore, ostarine and other SARMs ought to be avoided. They could turn out to be nothing worse than a waste of money, but they might even damage health, as the one case of liver toxicity showed.

Detox Supplements

Detoxing, the craze for ridding our bodies of toxins, or "cleansing", has swept the land. The idea is that toxins build up, and that by going through a special intervention that includes elements of fasting, vegetarian diet, drinking lemon water or other concoctions, and taking special detox supplements, we can purge toxins from our bodies and thus get healthier and even lose weight.

Unfortunately, the nature of these toxins usually goes unspecified. Furthermore, the human body has its own detoxification system, mainly the liver and the enzymes in it, so any toxins that are present can be eliminated. For example, the liver metabolizes drugs in this way to eliminate them from the body.

Going through a detox procedure or taking a detox supplement will do nothing to speed the process of ridding any putative toxins from the body. They're a waste of money, and the entire concept of detox or cleansing is bogus. Anecdotally, several people I know reported feeling ill while doing a "cleanse".

Toxins can be real, heavy metals and organic substances like the endocrine disruptor BPA being two that can cause genuine problems. Buildup of enough heavy metals, such as lead, cadmium, or mercury, could necessitate medical treatment; BPA may be rather quickly eliminated by the body so long as exposure to them is avoided. But in any case, detox supplements won't help you with either.

Fluoride

Hardly anyone takes fluoride supplements, fortunately, but unfortunately, your local government may force you to take it, since they add it to drinking water in many places. Toothpaste also contains fluoride, and you may ingest a certain amount of it that way. The label on a tube of toothpaste reads, "If more than is used for brushing is accidentally swallowed, get medical help or contact a Poison Control Center right way."

Fluoride is a poison, and putting it into the water amounts to medicating you without your consent, a clear breach of medical ethics.

Fluoride is not a required nutrient. We don't need it. It probably isn't even very effective against tooth decay.

Prolonged exposure to fluoride can damage the brain, and it's been linked to lower intelligence.[21] This seems particularly likely to cause harm in children, whose brains are developing. One of the authors of a report on fluoride and IQ likened it to "lead, mercury, and other poisons that cause chemical brain drain."

Fluoride has been linked to low testosterone and reduced sperm quality.[22] It's associated with a host of other problems, including thyroid disease, endocrine disruption, and cardiovascular disease. Fluoride can poison mitochondria, leading to chronic fatigue.

Since fluoride is not a required nutrient, and it has the potential to cause so many problems, and isn't even very effective against tooth decay, avoid it. Use bottled or filtered water; note that not all water filters remove fluoride. Check to see whether the water in your area is fluoridated. Personally, I also avoid fluoridated toothpaste; you can find non-fluoridated toothpaste fairly easily.

Supplements to Avoid – Key Points

- Calcium, iron, and copper should be avoided, yet they're in multivitamins
- Antioxidant vitamins may blunt the health effects of exercise
- Still, there can be reasons to take vitamin C

- Stay away from designer steroids, peptides, growth hormone promoters, and SARMs
- Detox supplements don't work
- Fluoride is poison.

10: The Dangers of Prescription Drugs and the Safety of Supplements

Mainstream medicine often warns that supplements can be dangerous, that they're unregulated and over-the-counter, and that people should be wary of them. While one should of course be cognizant of everything one puts into one's body, supplements have a good safety record. Mainstream medicine and the drugs it prescribes by the bucket-load are the real sources of dangerous substances.

Drug deaths now outnumber deaths in traffic accidents, according to an analysis in the Los Angeles Times.[1] Most of those deaths are driven by overdoses in prescription narcotics, such as oxycontin. The death total was more than 37,000.

A report from the Institute of Medicine suggested that medical errors resulted in an estimated 44,000 to 98,000 deaths annually in the U.S.[2] Many of these deaths are driven by medication errors, such as giving the wrong medication. While some reports have cast doubt on the magnitude of deaths, others say that the Institute of Medicine figures are not exaggerated.[3]

Patients who stay in hospitals can acquire infections there. As of 2011, there were an estimated annual 722,000 hospital-acquired infections, and approximately 10% of patients who got infections died during their hospital stay.[4]

Writing in the BMJ, Danish professor of psychiatry Peter Gøtzsche argues, "Psychiatric drugs are responsible for the deaths of more than half a million people aged 65 and older each year in the Western world, as I show below. Their benefits would need to be colossal to justify this, but they are minimal."[5] He estimates that three classes of drugs, antipsychotics, benzodiazepines and similar drugs (anti-anxiety drugs), and antidepressants cause excess mortality of 1, 1, and 2% respectively, and that when the U.S. and the European Union are combined, results in 539,000 deaths a year.

Gøtzsche also believes that most of these drugs do little good, and that "we could stop almost all psychotropic drugs without causing harm—by dropping all antidepressants, ADHD drugs, and dementia drugs (as the small effects are probably the result of unblinding bias) and using only a fraction of the antipsychotics and benzodiazepines we currently use. This would lead to healthier and more long lived populations. Because psychotropic drugs are immensely harmful when used long term, they should almost exclusively be used in acute situations and always with a firm plan for tapering off, which can be difficult for many patients."

While others disagree with him on the magnitude of the harms of psychiatric drugs, it seems clear that they have the potential for serious harm.

Daniel F. Kripke, M.D., a professor of psychiatry, has estimated that sleeping pills result in a large number of excess deaths.[6] He and colleagues note that 6 to 10% of American adults took a drug for poor sleep in 2010. Patients who had any prescription for a hypnotic (sleeping pill) had an increased risk of death, even when prescribed less than 18 pills a year. People taking more than 132 doses a year had a more than 5-fold increased risk of death. Cancer rates also increased about 35% in those taking the highest doses. In the statistical analysis, patients taking hypnotics were matched with controls who had the same condition but did not take hypnotics, leading to greater confidence that hypnotics (and not some other factor such as pre-existing illness) were behind the difference in death rates.

As of 2009, there were approximately 4.6 million emergency room visits connected to taking drugs, and of these, almost 50% were because of adverse effects from taking drugs as prescribed.[7]

Statins are widely prescribed drugs that lower cholesterol for alleged protection against heart attacks, and they come with a raft of side effects, including muscle pain and memory loss. More than 25% of Americans over the age of 45 use them.[8] Statins are relatively ineffective, and what little effect they have is not due to lowering cholesterol, which plays little if any role in atherosclerosis. Statins are associated with increased risk of cancer with long-term use, as well as diabetes. They may actually increase heart failure and atherosclerosis by depleting vitamin K2 and coenzyme Q10, and inhibiting the production of important antioxidant proteins.[9] Statins decrease testosterone in men.[10] Yet annual drug company revenue for statins is around $30 billion, and pharmaceutical companies have convinced doctors that they need to prescribe them to huge numbers of people.

In contrast to prescription drugs, Dr. Andrew Saul, writing for the Orthomolecular News Service, and citing the U.S. National Poison Data System, states that in 2015, there were "zero deaths from *any* supplement."[11] There were no deaths from vitamins, none from minerals, none from amino acids, and none from any herbal supplement.

Yet, mainstream medicine wants us to believe that supplements are dangerous, when clearly, their own products and services leave a lot to be desired. While some supplements could cause harm, especially when used wrongly, the fact of no deaths means that they appear to be far safer than prescription drugs or hospital stays. Hospitalization generally represents a more extreme measure for seriously ill people; while decreasing the chances of harm from staying in the hospital should be an urgent task, it's perhaps not surprising that patients can be seriously harmed in a hospital. Prescription drugs are another matter, because many are prescribed for non-serious illness, and in fact, there may not be very good reasons at all for prescribing many of them, as Peter Gøtzsche argues in the case of psychiatric drugs, and Daniel Kripke argues for sleeping pills.

Comparing the potential toxicity of the anti-anxiety supplement theanine with that of prescription anti-anxiety drugs such as benzodiazepines hardly even seems fair, so lopsided is the result. To my knowledge, theanine has never harmed much less killed anyone, but overdoses and other misadventures from tranquilizers are common. Similar arguments could be made regarding melatonin for sleep versus prescription sleeping pills.

You should always respect the power of anything you put in your body, whether that's food, drink, supplements, or drugs. One reason that certain drugs must be legally prescribed by a doctor is the potential for harm, with the doctor making a considered judgment whether prescribing the drug will result in greater benefit than harm. Yet it's estimated that in 2016, 4.27 billion prescriptions were filled in the U.S. – and that's at the retail level only.[12] Clearly, doctors are prescribing lots of drugs, and it would be hubris to assume that every one of those billions of prescriptions were for treatment of genuine illness for which nothing but a drug would do.

Prescription drugs are huge business. Global revenue for the pharmaceutical industry for 2015 was an estimated $1,072 billion, of which the North American market was nearly half.[13] There's a lot at stake in the drug biz, and drug companies will protect their sales at all costs. The stupendous sales of statin drugs accounts for much of the continued disparagement of dietary fat, in my view, despite emerging and good evidence that cholesterol levels have little if anything to do with atherosclerotic heart disease. While supplements may put only the smallest of dents in Big Pharma revenue, the interests of drug companies, doctors, and scientists alike align to disparage supplements and promote the use of prescription drugs.

11: Diet, Exercise, and Lifestyle

The supplements discussed in this book offer a range of benefits and effects, from marginal to lifesaving, depending on starting state of health, deficiencies, and other factors. Ideally, they should be used as an adjunct to a healthy lifestyle, and not depended on to work miracles on their own. If you don't eat, exercise, and sleep right, the health effects of adding any supplement may be minimal to non-existent. Healthy practices should be the basis of your health, and in this chapter, I'll briefly discuss what those healthy practices are, as always in my humble opinion.

My philosophy on diet and exercise boils down to this:

Cut the carbs and sugar, and lift weights.

The rest is commentary.

Diet

The food you eat can make or break your health, and with it your ability to add or maintain muscle, to have normal testosterone levels, and to live a long life free of disease. Diet is arguably the most important part of a healthy lifestyle, but what constitutes a healthy diet is controversial. Starting decades ago, health authorities began recommending that people cut the fat out of their diets with the aim of preventing heart disease, even though the evidence that dietary fat caused heart disease was scanty and of low quality. That must have been the first time in human history that anyone thought fat was undesirable or unhealthy; humans have always sought out fatty food.

That brings us to a principle of food and health that we can use to determine what is and is not good for us, the principle being that the foods that our ancestors ate and thrived on for thousands or millions of years is likely to be healthy. Determining exactly what those foods are, and in what proportions, can be a difficult proposition, and what people ate likely varied greatly in different times and places. However, we can more readily use that principle to determine what they *didn't* eat, since they had no access to much of what we eat in the modern age.

Our modern, processed foods contribute to the diseases of civilization, such as obesity, heart disease, cancer, and diabetes, and are probably the most important factor. Processed food is perhaps better called industrial food, since it's made on an industrial scale using methods that weren't available to our ancestors.

The three main ingredients of industrial foods that cause illness and premature aging are:

- Vegetable oils
- Sugar
- White flour.

Vegetable oils

Vegetable oils are made by an industrial process from seeds, and hence are better called industrial seed oils. A few of them have been used in small quantities in history, but modern manufacturing methods in the early 20th century allowed oils to be extracted from plants that hadn't been used before and which contained little oil, such as soybeans, corn, and canola.

Seed oils contain high proportions of omega-6 fatty acids, and little omega-3, so their consumption leads to an imbalance of these fats in our diet, with the consequences that that entails. Omega-6 fats cause cancer and heart disease, and are highly suspect in diabetes and other illnesses, especially those with an inflammatory component.

The invention of hydrogenation allowed seed oils to be made into other products, such as margarine and shortening; these are loaded with another form of fat, trans fat, which are not found in nature. (Except in very small amounts, and the natural forms differ from industrial forms.)

Virtually all modern processed food and fast food uses industrial seed oils. They're used in breads, pastries, and frozen foods; in deep fryers at your local fast food restaurant; in salad dressings and margarine. For the sake of your health you should avoid them and anything made with them. The implications here are fairly drastic: to stay healthy and lean, you should avoid almost all processed and fast food, and eat whole, unprocessed food only.

The oils to be avoided include:

- Corn
- Soy

- Canola
- Peanut
- Sunflower
- Safflower
- Cottonseed.

Note that olive oil and coconut oil are not industrial seed oils, are healthy, and may be used freely. For cooking, you can use both of these, as well as butter, ghee, and animal fat including non-hydrogenized lard.

Sugar

Sugar in some form or other has been known for thousands of years, but advances in production starting in the 18th century led to vastly increased consumption. In the early 19th century, sugar consumption was as little as a few pounds a year per person, but by the early 21st century that rose to as much as 100 pounds per person per year. While that figure has decreased somewhat in recent years as people get the message that all that sugar isn't healthy, recent figures show the average person consumes 60 to 80 pounds of sugar annually, and that figure doesn't include fruit juice, a large source.[1]

Eating sugar in more than minimal amounts leads to obesity, diabetes, heart disease, and cancer, the modern diseases of civilization. As humans have overcome the infectious diseases that have plagued them since time immemorial, now we're faced with degenerative diseases, and those are mostly caused by diet, sugar playing a large role. The fact that sugar rots teeth should give us a clue as to its other health effects.

Health authorities used to think of sugar as benign, although most parents knew better, and sugar consumption increased with the advent of the craze for low-fat eating. The switch to higher sugar consumption is one of the main factors leading to the obesity epidemic.

Evidence points to sugar as a cause of heart disease.

A study published in the Journal of the American Medical Association found highly positive and graded correlations between sugar intake and death from cardiovascular (heart) disease (CVD).[2] Comparing quintiles (fifths) of sugar intake, the highest consumers had more than double the risk of dying from CVD. In the highest consumers, who ate >25% of their calories as sugar, *the risk nearly tripled.* Those who consumed >10% but <25% of calories as sugar, had 30% increased risk of death.

Most adults that this study looked at, 71% of them, consumed more than 10% of calories as added sugar, and around 10% of them consumed more than 25% of calories as added sugar.

The heart disease risk may be underestimated, when you compare high consumers of sugar to people who consume no sugar at all. Since over 70% of adults consume more than 10% of calories as sugar, people who eat zero sugar must be hard to find, at least enough for a study.

Dietary sugar is associated with hypertension – high blood pressure, and that's independent of weight gain. This may occur due to high levels of insulin, with subsequent increase in body water. Insulin is an anti-diuretic: it increases the retention of fluid. Salt is only minimally related to hypertension. The correlation between processed foods and hypertension arises not from salt, but sugar.[3]

Sugar causes levels of triglycerides to increase, and triglycerides are associated with CVD; it also causes HDL cholesterol to drop; both of those are probably just markers for increased insulin resistance; it also increases inflammatory markers, which are associated with CVD.

It's likely that all of the above mechanisms and effects are due to insulin resistance.

Sugar (sucrose) is a molecule made of a fructose and a glucose molecule linked together. Hence, sugar is 50% glucose, 50% fructose. High-fructose corn syrup, which is increasingly used in place of sugar, is 45% glucose and 55% fructose – it's not that different.

Fructose seems to be the bad element here. A high intake of fructose leads to hyperlipidemia (high fat in the blood) and to insulin resistance.[4]

Franceso Facchini and Gerald Reaven, both at Stanford University, studied a group of 290 apparently healthy men and classified them according to tertiles (thirds) of insulin resistance. He then followed them for a number of years and looked at the type and number of diseases they got, including hypertension, CVD, diabetes, cancer, and stroke.

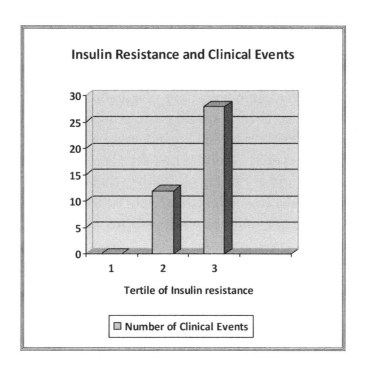

Those in the lowest third of insulin resistance remained perfectly healthy, with zero cases of disease. Those in the highest third had 28 "events" of heart disease, cancer, stroke, and the rest. Insulin resistance may explain how and why sugar is associated with heart disease.

Sugar is also associated with diabetes, obesity, and probably cancer. Higher consumption of soda and other sugar-sweetened beverages (SSBs) is associated with far greater odds of obesity.[5]

Over 75% of processed food in the U.S. contains added sugar. The worst offenders are the SSBs – soda, sports drinks, and fruit juices – as well as desserts, candy, cake, and pastries. But they add sugar to almost everything.

Again, we see why you must avoid processed food to be lean and healthy.

The American Heart Association recommends men consume no more than 9 teaspoons of sugar daily, women 6 teaspoons. (One soda contains about 10 teaspoons of sugar.) In my view, even that is too much and could lead to obesity and illness; however, if you have no other health problems, are not overweight, and are physically active, that amount may cause little trouble. If you are overweight or have health problems, all sugar should be religiously avoided.

Refined Carbohydrates

Carbohydrate sources that have been milled or otherwise refined include the classic example of white flour, and others like white rice and corn meal. Fiber and other nutrients have been removed from refined carbohydrates; that allows for longer storage and makes them a quintessentially industrial food.

Refined carbohydrates are associated with much greater risk of obesity, heart disease, diabetes, and probably cancer.[6]

Probably the main reason refined carbohydrates work such havoc is by spiking blood glucose (blood sugar); they have a high glycemic index, meaning a high capacity for raising blood sugar. When blood sugar spikes, insulin rises, and the energy from these foods tends to be stored as fat. Classically, this leads to a crash in blood sugar in a few hours, and ravenous hunger follows, leading to a vicious cycle of high and low blood sugar and insulin, fat storage, and ultimately obesity.

Foods that are high in refined carbohydrates include:

- Bread
- Pasta
- Tortillas
- White rice
- Breakfast cereal
- Pizza

Anyone who wants to lose weight and preserve health should avoid these. I gave them up years ago and have never felt better.

What to eat

Just about everyone eats a typical American diet loaded with vegetable oils, sugar, and refined carbohydrates, and it's no coincidence that the current combined rate of overweight and obesity is about 70%. If you don't want to be a victim of modern processed food, what do you eat?

Changing your diet from modern industrial garbage to one that promotes and supports health requires a sea change in attitude. No longer can you just zip over the local fast-food joint to pick up lunch or dinner. You can't stroll down the center aisles of supermarkets and load your cart with sodas and frozen pizza. You will need to choose your food carefully, and you will need to prepare much of it at home.

Eat minimally processed, whole foods, such as:

- Meat
- Eggs
- Cheese
- Yogurt – made with whole milk, and unsweetened
- Butter and cream
- Vegetables and leafy greens
- Fruit
- Nuts

A few caveats.

1. Those wanting to lose weight should avoid starchy vegetables such as potatoes and sweet potatoes. If you're lean and active, go ahead and eat them. Personally, I eat as few carbohydrates as possible, but not everyone shares the need or desire. Note however that the typical American eats 50% of his or her food as carbohydrates, and the typical American is overweight or obese. While not everyone needs to avoid all starches or carbohydrates, any restriction of carbohydrates is beneficial.

2. Fruit is high in sugar and likewise, those wanting to lose weight should only eat minimal if any fruit. The fruits that our ancestors ate, and only in season, were not like those of today, which have been bred to be bags of sugar. Dried fruit (e.g. raisins, apricots) contains an especially large amount of sugar.

3. Nuts are high in calories and in omega-6 fats. Don't go overboard on them; they can cause weight gain.

4. At the supermarket, shop around the outer aisles of the store and avoid the inner aisles, which is where they keep the highly processed food.
5. Drink non-caloric beverages, such as water, coffee, and tea. If you drink alcohol, don't drink beer or anything sweetened.

Exercise and Its Myths

Exercise remains a cornerstone of good health. Your level of physical fitness is highly correlated with life expectancy, and being sedentary is associated with much higher mortality risks. Everyone should exercise, and generally speaking, the more you exercise the better. (Although as with anything, one can take exercise too far – see under marathon running.)

However, there are some myths associated with exercise, myths that can actually harm people's health, more so because they are so widespread. The main two harmful exercise myths are:

1. Exercise helps you lose weight.
2. Aerobic exercise is a uniquely beneficial form of exercise.

Let's demolish these myths, show what exercise can and cannot do, and what a beneficial exercise program looks like.

Weight Loss

Exercise, that is, garden-variety aerobic exercise, the kind most people do, has a terrible record at weight loss. Many studies have shown little to no effect of exercise at helping people lose weight when not accompanied by dietary changes.[7] A review of studies stated conclusively, "Our results show that isolated aerobic exercise is not an effective weight loss therapy in these patients [overweight and obese]."

Yet everyone believes that exercise does. In part, this myth is promulgated by food and beverage companies, who do not want people to believe that their products cause obesity. Thus, they send a message of "balance", and that if you're overweight it's your own fault because you're lazy.

Another facet of this exercise myth concerns burning of calories, the idea being that if you spend an hour exercising and use, say, 300 calories, you'll lose weight. There are several problems with this idea. One is that exercise just doesn't burn all that many calories. The average adult man needs perhaps 1500 calories a day just to maintain himself without weight loss and to stay alive; he needs that much if he does nothing more than sit all day. In comparison, running 5 miles, which most people would consider a very vigorous workout, burns about 500 calories. Walking for 30 minutes consumes around 200. Those figures don't add appreciably to the total number of calories burned.

Exercise also makes you hungry, so after your exercise session, you're likely to eat more than if you hadn't exercised, enough to partly or wholly negate the calories burned in exercise, or even worse, you might eat enough to *gain* weight.

Furthermore, it's trivially easy to eat enough to more than make up for calories burned. If you go out and run those 5 miles, and then get a fancy coffee drink afterwards, you will have consumed more calories than you burned. People famously like to "treat" themselves with a snack or some other food/drink reward after exercise, and those treats abolish the calories burned.

Exercise promotes health, but diet is by far the most important factor in weight loss.

Aerobic Exercise

For several decades now, mainstream health and fitness authorities have recommended aerobic exercise, also known as endurance exercise or "cardio", as the best way to exercise and get fit. And Americans have been following that advice, and now exercise more than ever.

As with the universal recommendation to eat low-fat foods, the advice to do aerobics was given starting right around the time that the obesity epidemic got going. Many knowledgeable people believe that the low-fat craze and the obesity epidemic are intimately related. What about aerobics – could that have contributed to the obesity epidemic too? Could be. For one thing, people exercising aerobically believe that it will help them lose weight, when as we've seen, evidence says otherwise, so they might be complacent about what they eat.

As humans get older, they lose muscle at a predictable rate if they don't do anything about it. Between ages 50 and 70, most people will have lost 30% of their muscle mass, and then another 20% or so to age 80, a full half of all muscle being lost by that age. The loss of muscle is largely responsible for the fact that most people gain fat as they get older, even when eating the same quantity and quality of food as when they were younger; muscle burns more energy than other tissues, so when it's lost or replaced, total metabolic rate declines, and if food intake doesn't also decline, fat gain ensues.

Aerobic exercise does next to nothing to fight muscle loss. Walking is probably the most common form of aerobic exercise that people engage in, and if someone did nothing but walk, they will typically still lose 4 to 6 pounds of lean mass every decade, along with a decline of 2 to 3% in resting metabolic rate, essentially no different than if that person was completely sedentary.

Aerobics, or at least walking, could lead to fat gain by allowing the loss of muscle mass.

While aerobic exercise promotes health and prevents cardiovascular disease and cancer, it's not the only form of exercise that does so. Aerobics is based on the idea that a relatively slow-pace at a steady-state and a longer duration of activity have unique health benefits. But other forms of exercise, notably high intensity interval training (HIIT), and strength training, also improve health markers. In particular, HIIT improves health markers in an extraordinarily small amount of time, with sprint cyclers getting as fit as aerobic exercisers in only 10% of the time. Furthermore, both strength training and HIIT are less likely to lead to the sort of overuse injuries in knees, hips, and feet that are so often seen with aerobics.

The two myths of exercise, that it causes weight loss and that you must do aerobic exercise to be healthy, harm people by lulling them into a sense of complacency regarding their weight and their diet, and by doing nothing to stem the tide of muscle loss in aging.

Combining what I've written so far in this chapter, attention to a healthy diet low in industrial food, and an exercise program that combines strength training (lifting weights) and high intensity interval training, are your best bets to become and stay lean and healthy, and to give you your best shot at a long life. The current paradigm of low-fat eating and aerobic exercise is suboptimal at best. As this is meant only as a brief summary, for more complete explanations, as well as exercise and diet programs, see my books *Muscle Up* and *Stop the Clock*.

Grazing and Fasting

Besides the type and amount of food you eat, there's also the matter of when you eat it.

The most robust (non-genetic) intervention known for prolonging the lifespan of lab animals is calorie restriction (CR). Animals that have their food restricted from 10 to 50% of that of fully-fed animals live much longer, in some cases 50% longer.

Many theories have arisen as to why CR increases lifespan. One theory is that CR results in less fat tissue, and that this is crucial to longer life. Other theories have to do with repressed insulin signaling and/or increased autophagy, the cellular self-cleansing process that rids cells of junk. Likely all of these theories are related to each other mechanistically. I like to focus on autophagy, because this is a marker within our control to some extent.

Aging is characterized by a decline in the amount and amplitude of autophagy, which allows increased amounts of cellular damage and junk to accumulate.

Autophagy is strongly cyclical, rising and falling over periods of hours and days. Eating strongly decreases autophagy, and fasting increases it. If aging means less autophagy and more damage accumulation, and fasting increases autophagy, then fasting fights aging.

In fact, intermittent fasting may be one of the most potent anti-aging strategies available.

Now, if we eat all the time, we never enter the fasting state and never up-regulate autophagy.

Eating constantly or every few hours, or "grazing" as it's called, is one of the most potent pro-aging actions available.

Stop eating all the time.

Grazing is one of the most asinine "health" interventions of modern times.

How often does eating have to be to constitute "all the time"?

To answer that, it's helpful to look at what people did in the old days — say, about 40 years ago, before the obesity epidemic started. Or even more so, before the era of industrial processed food and cheap fast-food restaurants or even refrigerators. It was common for people to fast for 12 hours daily, from dinner in the evening until breakfast the next morning. Many mothers often told their children, "Better eat your dinner because there won't be anything until breakfast." My mom did anyway.

One factor that doesn't get enough attention in obesity is the frequency with which we eat. When we eat constantly, insulin never drops by much, and so lipolysis, the exit of fat from fat cells, can't take place.

Contrary to popular belief, energy expenditure has not decreased in recent years and is similar in modern people to that of wild, non-overweight, mammals, and Westerners seem to expend the same amount of energy as hunter-gatherers.

Hunter-gatherers of course eat different food from Westerners, but they also don't eat all the time.

Our distant ancestors way back in the 1960s had a far lower rate of obesity while still eating, in general, lots of crappy food. They weren't interested in "health food", but largely managed to keep obesity at bay anyway.

The lesson is clear, to stay lean and/or lose weight, **stop eating all the time.**

Current mainstream advice on losing weight states that we need to eat constantly in order to keep our metabolism up. In fact, the admonition to eat constantly, or graze, is the kind of BS weight-loss advice that's perpetuating the obesity epidemic.

You cannot lose weight by eating more often, even if those meals and snacks are smaller. Not only will someone who eats constantly fail to lose much weight, but he'll promote aging and the diseases that go with it.

Drop the snacks too.

Other Lifestyle Factors

Sleep is arguably the most important of the other lifestyle factors for health. Poor sleep can ruin health, and is often a symptom of other problems. Previously in this book, I touched on the importance of artificial light in hampering sleep; besides light, alcohol, caffeine, and stress can all cause poor sleep. If you often don't sleep well, you should figure out what's causing that and fix it for the sake of your health.

Other important lifestyle factors that can harm health include:

- Stress
- Social isolation
- Alcohol use
- Use of pornography
- Being sedentary – even if you exercise at other times

Conversely, religious practice, friends and family life, social involvement, leisure-time physical activity, and being productive can all improve health, both physical and mental.

Hopefully, this brief tour of diet, exercise, and other lifestyle factors in relation to health has placed the role of supplements in perspective. You won't achieve optimal health merely by taking supplements; while they can be a big help, you must heed these other factors too.

About the Author

P. D. (Dennis) Mangan is the author of 7 books on health and fitness, and is the proprietor of the website Rogue Health and Fitness, at http://roguehealthandfitness.com/. He lives in California.

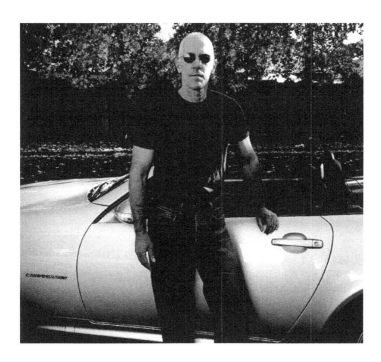

Notes

Chapter 1

[1] Martínez Steele E, Baraldi LG, Louzada MLDC, et al Ultra-processed foods and added sugars in the US diet: evidence from a nationally representative cross-sectional study BMJ Open 2016;6:e009892. doi: 10.1136/bmjopen-2015-009892
[2] https://www.scientificamerican.com/article/the-hidden-harm-of-antidepressants/

Chapter 2

[1] PD Mangan, *Muscle Up*, Phalanx Press, 2015
[2] Bandegan, Arash, et al. "Indicator Amino Acid–Derived Estimate of Dietary Protein Requirement for Male Bodybuilders on a Nontraining Day Is Several-Fold Greater than the Current Recommended Dietary Allowance." The Journal of Nutrition (2017): jn236331.
[3] Lemon, P. W., et al. "Protein requirements and muscle mass/strength changes during intensive training in novice bodybuilders." *Journal of Applied Physiology* 73.2 (1992): 767-775.
[4] Norton, Layne E., et al. "The leucine content of a complete meal directs peak activation but not duration of skeletal muscle protein synthesis and mammalian target of rapamycin signaling in rats." *The Journal of nutrition* 139.6 (2009): 1103-1109.
[5] Hennesy, Maggie, Leucine: Where whey protein gets its magic. http://www.nutraingredients-usa.com/Markets/Leucine-Where-whey-protein-gets-its-magic
[6] Zemel, Michael B., and Antje Bruckbauer. "Effects of a leucine and pyridoxine-containing nutraceutical on fat oxidation, and oxidative and inflammatory stress in overweight and obese subjects." *Nutrients* 4.6 (2012): 529-541.
[7] Frestedt, Joy L., et al. "A whey-protein supplement increases fat loss and spares lean muscle in obese subjects: a randomized human clinical study." *Nutrition & Metabolism* 5.1 (2008): 8.
[8] Hansen, Mette, et al. "Effect of whey protein hydrolysate on performance and recovery of top-class orienteering runners." *International journal of sport nutrition and exercise metabolism* 25.2 (2015): 97-109.
[9] Breen, Leigh, and Stuart M. Phillips. "Skeletal muscle protein metabolism in the elderly: Interventions to counteract the 'anabolic resistance' of ageing." *Nutrition & Metabolism* 8.1 (2011): 68.
[10] Bechshøft, Rasmus Leidesdorff, et al. "Improved skeletal muscle mass and strength after heavy strength training in very old individuals." *Experimental Gerontology* (2017).
[11] Valerio, Alessandra, Giuseppe D'Antona, and Enzo Nisoli. "Branched-chain amino acids, mitochondrial biogenesis, and healthspan: an evolutionary perspective." *Aging (Albany NY)* 3.5 (2011): 464-478.

[12] Schoenfeld, Brad Jon, Alan Albert Aragon, and James W. Krieger. "The effect of protein timing on muscle strength and hypertrophy: a meta-analysis." *Journal of the International Society of Sports Nutrition* 10.1 (2013): 53.
[13] Groen, Bart, et al. "Protein ingestion before sleep improves postexercise overnight recovery." *Medicine and science in sports and exercise* 44.8 (2012): 1560-1569.
[14] Bauer, Jürgen M., et al. "Effects of a vitamin D and leucine-enriched whey protein nutritional supplement on measures of sarcopenia in older adults, the PROVIDE study: a randomized, double-blind, placebo-controlled trial." *Journal of the American Medical Directors Association* 16.9 (2015): 740-747.
[15] Evans, William J. "Skeletal muscle loss: cachexia, sarcopenia, and inactivity." *The American Journal of Clinical Nutrition* 91.4 (2010): 1123S-1127S.
[16] McWhirter, Janet P., and Christopher R. Pennington. "Incidence and recognition of malnutrition in hospital." *Bmj* 308.6934 (1994): 945-948.
[17] Brown, Rex O., et al. "Comparison of specialized and standard enteral formulas in trauma patients." *Pharmacotherapy: The Journal of Human Pharmacology and Drug Therapy* 14.3 (1994): 314-320.
[18] Corti, Maria-Chiara, et al. "Serum albumin level and physical disability as predictors of mortality in older persons." *Jama* 272.13 (1994): 1036-1042.
[19] MacLennan, W. J., P. Martin, and B. J. Mason. "Protein intake and serum albumin levels in the elderly." *Gerontology* 23.5 (1977): 360-367.
[20] Novak, Frantisek, et al. "Glutamine supplementation in serious illness: a systematic review of the evidence." *Critical care medicine* 30.9 (2002): 2022-2029.
[21] Gleeson, Michael. "Dosing and efficacy of glutamine supplementation in human exercise and sport training." *The Journal of Nutrition* 138.10 (2008): 2045S-2049S.
[22] Candow, Darren G., et al. "Effect of glutamine supplementation combined with resistance training in young adults." *European Journal of Applied Physiology* 86.2 (2001): 142-149.
[23] Smith, Gordon I., et al. "Dietary omega-3 fatty acid supplementation increases the rate of muscle protein synthesis in older adults: a randomized controlled trial." *The American journal of clinical nutrition* 93.2 (2011): 402-412.
[24] Smith, Gordon I., et al. "Omega-3 polyunsaturated fatty acids augment the muscle protein anabolic response to hyperinsulinaemia—hyperaminoacidaemia in healthy young and middle-aged men and women." *Clinical Science* 121.6 (2011): 267-278.
[25] Kim, Hyo Jeong, et al. "Studies on the safety of creatine supplementation." *Amino acids* 40.5 (2011): 1409-1418.
[26] Volek, Jeff S., et al. "Performance and muscle fiber adaptations to creatine supplementation and heavy resistance training." *Medicine and science in sports and exercise* 31 (1999): 1147-1156.
[27] Chrusch, Murray J., et al. "Creatine supplementation combined with resistance training in older men." *Medicine and science in sports and exercise* 33.12 (2001): 2111-2117.
[28] Bender, A., et al. "Creatine improves health and survival of mice." *Neurobiology of Aging* 29.9 (2008): 1404-1411.
[29] Gualano, Bruno, et al. "Exploring the therapeutic role of creatine supplementation." *Amino acids* 38.1 (2010): 31-44.
[30] Hultman, E., et al. "Muscle creatine loading in men." *Journal of applied physiology* 81.1 (1996): 232-237.
[31] Hultman, E., et al. "Muscle creatine loading in men." *Journal of applied*

physiology 81.1 (1996): 232-237

Chapter 3

[1] Harman, S. Mitchell, et al. "Longitudinal effects of aging on serum total and free testosterone levels in healthy men." *The Journal of Clinical Endocrinology & Metabolism* 86.2 (2001): 724-731.
[2] Andersson, Anna-Maria, et al. "Secular decline in male testosterone and sex hormone binding globulin serum levels in Danish population surveys." *The Journal of Clinical Endocrinology & Metabolism* 92.12 (2007): 4696-4705.
[3] Khaw, Kay-Tee, et al. "Endogenous testosterone and mortality due to all causes, cardiovascular disease, and cancer in men." *Circulation* 116.23 (2007): 2694-2701.
[4] Bhasin, Shalender, et al. "The effects of supraphysiologic doses of testosterone on muscle size and strength in normal men." *N Engl j Med* 1996.335 (1996): 1-7.
[5] Prasad, A. S., et al. "Zinc deficiency in elderly patients." *Nutrition (Burbank, Los Angeles County, Calif.)* 9.3 (1992): 218-224.
[6] Dardenne, Mireille, et al. "Restoration of the thymus in aging mice by in vivo zinc supplementation." *Clinical immunology and immunopathology* 66.2 (1993): 127-135.
[7] Haase, Hajo, and Lothar Rink. "The immune system and the impact of zinc during aging." *Immunity & Ageing* 6.1 (2009): 9.
[8] Prasad, Ananda S., et al. "Zinc in cancer prevention." *Nutrition and cancer* 61.6 (2009): 879-887.
[9] Gonzalez, Alejandro, et al. "Zinc intake from supplements and diet and prostate cancer." *Nutrition and cancer* 61.2 (2009): 206-215.
[10] Haase, Hajo, and Lothar Rink. "The immune system and the impact of zinc during aging." *Immunity & Ageing* 6.1 (2009): 9.
[11] Prasad, Ananda S., et al. "Zinc status and serum testosterone levels of healthy adults." *Nutrition* 12.5 (1996): 344-348.
[12] Koehler, K., et al. "Serum testosterone and urinary excretion of steroid hormone metabolites after administration of a high-dose zinc supplement." *European journal of clinical nutrition* 63.1 (2009): 65-70.
[13] Wilborn, Colin D., et al. "Effects of zinc magnesium aspartate (ZMA) supplementation on training adaptations and markers of anabolism and catabolism." *Journal of the International Society of Sports Nutrition* 1.2 (2004): 12.
[14] Wegmüller, Rita, et al. "Zinc absorption by young adults from supplemental zinc citrate is comparable with that from zinc gluconate and higher than from zinc oxide." *The Journal of nutrition* 144.2 (2014): 132-136.
[15] King, Dana E., et al. "Dietary magnesium and C-reactive protein levels." *Journal of the American College of Nutrition* 24.3 (2005): 166-171.
[16] Rosanoff, Andrea. "The high heart health value of drinking-water magnesium." *Medical hypotheses* 81.6 (2013): 1063-1065.
[17] Peacock, James M., et al. "Serum magnesium and risk of sudden cardiac death in the Atherosclerosis Risk in Communities (ARIC) Study." *American heart journal* 160.3 (2010): 464-470.
[18] Joosten, Michel M., et al. "Urinary and plasma magnesium and risk of ischemic heart disease." *The American journal of clinical nutrition* 97.6 (2013): 1299-1306.
[19] Derom, Marie-Laure, et al. "Magnesium and depression: a systematic review." *Nutritional neuroscience* 16.5 (2013): 191-206.
[20] Barragán-Rodríguez, Lazaro, Martha Rodríguez-Morán, and Fernando Guerrero-

Romero. "Efficacy and safety of oral magnesium supplementation in the treatment of depression in the elderly with type 2 diabetes: a randomized, equivalent trial." *Magnesium Research* 21.4 (2008): 218-223.

[21] Eby, George A., and Karen L. Eby. "Rapid recovery from major depression using magnesium treatment." *Medical hypotheses* 67.2 (2006): 362-370.

[22] Maggio, M., et al. "Magnesium and anabolic hormones in older men." *International journal of andrology* 34.6pt2 (2011).

[23] Cinar, Vedat, et al. "Effects of magnesium supplementation on testosterone levels of athletes and sedentary subjects at rest and after exhaustion." *Biological trace element research* 140.1 (2011): 18-23.

[24] Brilla, Lorraine R., and Timothy F. Haley. "Effect of magnesium supplementation on strength training in humans." *Journal of the American College of Nutrition* 11.3 (1992): 326-329.

[25] http://www.magnesiumeducation.com/how-much-mg

[26] Walker, Ann F., et al. "Mg citrate found more bioavailable than other Mg preparations in a randomised, double-blind study." *Magnesium research* 16.3 (2003): 183-191.

[27] Cormio, Luigi, et al. "Oral L-citrulline supplementation improves erection hardness in men with mild erectile dysfunction." *Urology* 77.1 (2011): 119-122.

[28] Stanislavov, R., and P. Rohdewald. "Sperm quality in men is improved by supplementation with a combination of L-arginine, L-citrullin, roburins and Pycnogenol®." *Minerva urologica e nefrologica= The Italian journal of urology and nephrology* 66.4 (2014): 217-223.

[29] BRUNINI, Tatiana MC, et al. "Diminished L-arginine bioavailability in hypertension." *Clinical science* 107.4 (2004): 391-397.

[30] Takeda, Kohei, et al. "Effects of citrulline supplementation on fatigue and exercise performance in mice." *Journal of nutritional science and vitaminology* 57.3 (2010): 246-250.

[31] Bendahan, D., et al. "Citrulline/malate promotes aerobic energy production in human exercising muscle." *British journal of sports medicine* 36.4 (2002): 282-289.

[32] Pérez-Guisado, Joaquín, and Philip M. Jakeman. "Citrulline malate enhances athletic anaerobic performance and relieves muscle soreness." *The Journal of Strength & Conditioning Research* 24.5 (2010): 1215-1222.

[33] Villareal, Dennis T., John O. Holloszy, and Wendy M. Kohrt. "Effects of DHEA replacement on bone mineral density and body composition in elderly women and men." *Clinical endocrinology* 53.5 (2000): 561-568.

[34] Morales, Arlene J., et al. "Effects of replacement dose of dehydroepiandrosterone in men and women of advancing age." *The Journal of Clinical Endocrinology & Metabolism* 78.6 (1994): 1360-1367.

[35] Panjari, Mary, et al. "The safety of 52 weeks of oral DHEA therapy for postmenopausal women." *Maturitas* 63.3 (2009): 240-245.

[36] Naghii, M. R., and S. Samman. "The effect of boron supplementation on its urinary excretion and selected cardiovascular risk factors in healthy male subjects." *Biological trace element research* 56.3 (1997): 273-286.

[37] Naghii, Mohammad Reza, et al. "Comparative effects of daily and weekly boron supplementation on plasma steroid hormones and proinflammatory cytokines." *Journal of trace elements in medicine and biology* 25.1 (2011): 54-58.

[38] Ferrando, Arny A., and Nancy R. Green. "The effect of boron supplementation on lean body mass, plasma testosterone levels, and strength in male bodybuilders." *International journal of sport nutrition* 3.2 (1993): 140-149.

[39] Balunas, Marcy J., et al. "Natural products as aromatase inhibitors." *Anti-Cancer Agents in Medicinal Chemistry (Formerly Current Medicinal Chemistry-Anti-Cancer Agents)* 8.6 (2008): 646-682.

[40] Eng, E. T., et al. "Anti-Aromatase Chemicals in Red Wine." *Annals of the New York Academy of Sciences* 963.1 (2002): 239-246.

[41] Kijima, Ikuko, et al. "Grape seed extract is an aromatase inhibitor and a suppressor of aromatase expression." *Cancer research* 66.11 (2006): 5960-5967.

[42] Bradlow, H. Leon, et al. "Effects of dietary indole-3-carbinol on estradiol metabolism and spontaneous mammary tumors in mice." *Carcinogenesis* 12.9 (1991): 1571-1574.

[43] Wehr, Elisabeth, et al. "Association of vitamin D status with serum androgen levels in men." *Clinical endocrinology* 73.2 (2010): 243-248.

[44] Pilz, S., et al. "Effect of vitamin D supplementation on testosterone levels in men." *Hormone and Metabolic Research* 43.03 (2011): 223-225.

[45] Dording, Christina M., et al. "A Double-Blind, Randomized, Pilot Dose-Finding Study of Maca Root (L. Meyenii) for the Management of SSRI-Induced Sexual Dysfunction." *CNS Neuroscience & Therapeutics* 14.3 (2008): 182-191.

[46] Gonzales, Gustavo F., et al. "Lepidium meyenii (Maca) improved semen parameters in adult men." *Asian Journal of Andrology* 3.4 (2001): 301-304.

[47] Gonzales, Gustavo F., et al. "Red maca (Lepidium meyenii) reduced prostate size in rats." *Reproductive Biology and Endocrinology* 3.1 (2005): 5.

Chapter 4

[1] Simopoulos, Artemis P. "Omega-3 fatty acids in health and disease and in growth and development." *The American journal of clinical nutrition* 54.3 (1991): 438-463.

[2] Leaf, Alexander, and Peter C. Weber. "Cardiovascular effects of n-3 fatty acids." *New England Journal of Medicine* 318.9 (1988): 549-557.

[3] Iso, Hiroyasu, et al. "Intake of fish and n3 fatty acids and risk of coronary heart disease among Japanese." *Circulation* 113.2 (2006): 195-202.

[4] Harris, William S. "Omega-3 fatty acids and cardiovascular disease: a case for omega-3 index as a new risk factor." *Pharmacological research* 55.3 (2007): 217-223.

[5] Cockbain, A. J., G. J. Toogood, and M. A. Hull. "Omega-3 polyunsaturated fatty acids for the treatment and prevention of colorectal cancer." *Gut* (2011): gut-2010.

[6] https://www.drsinatra.com/debunking-the-cancer-myth-the-health-benefits-of-omega-3s-against-prostate-cancer/

[7] Zhao, L. G., et al. "Fish consumption and all-cause mortality: a meta-analysis of cohort studies." *European journal of clinical nutrition* 70.2 (2016): 155-161.

[8] Li, Fang, Xiaoqin Liu, and Dongfeng Zhang. "Fish consumption and risk of depression: a meta-analysis." *J Epidemiol Community Health* 70.3 (2016): 299-304.

[9] Nemets, Boris, Ziva Stahl, and R. H. Belmaker. "Addition of omega-3 fatty acid to maintenance medication treatment for recurrent unipolar depressive disorder." *American Journal of Psychiatry* 159.3 (2002): 477-479.

[10] Su, Kuan-Pin, et al. "Omega-3 fatty acids in major depressive disorder: a preliminary double-blind, placebo-controlled trial." *European Neuropsychopharmacology* 13.4 (2003): 267-271.
[11] Edwards, Rhian, et al. "Omega-3 polyunsaturated fatty acid levels in the diet and in red blood cell membranes of depressed patients." *Journal of affective disorders* 48.2 (1998): 149-155.
[12] Thies, Frank, et al. "Dietary supplementation with eicosapentaenoic acid, but not with other long-chain n– 3 or n– 6 polyunsaturated fatty acids, decreases natural killer cell activity in healthy subjects aged> 55 y." *The American journal of clinical nutrition* 73.3 (2001): 539-548.
[13] Daviglus, Martha L., et al. "Fish consumption and the 30-year risk of fatal myocardial infarction." *New England Journal of Medicine* 336.15 (1997): 1046-1053.

Chapter 5

[1] Simpson, S. J., and D. Raubenheimer. "Obesity: the protein leverage hypothesis." *obesity reviews* 6.2 (2005): 133-142.
[2] Paddon-Jones, Douglas, et al. "Protein, weight management, and satiety." *The American journal of clinical nutrition* 87.5 (2008): 1558S-1561S.
[3] Weigle, David S., et al. "A high-protein diet induces sustained reductions in appetite, ad libitum caloric intake, and body weight despite compensatory changes in diurnal plasma leptin and ghrelin concentrations." *The American journal of clinical nutrition* 82.1 (2005): 41-48.
[4] Frestedt, Joy L., et al. "A whey-protein supplement increases fat loss and spares lean muscle in obese subjects: a randomized human clinical study." *Nutrition & Metabolism* 5.1 (2008): 8.
[5] Verreijen, Amely M., et al. "A high whey protein–, leucine-, and vitamin D– enriched supplement preserves muscle mass during intentional weight loss in obese older adults: a double-blind randomized controlled trial." *The American journal of clinical nutrition* 101.2 (2015): 279-286.
[6] Loenneke, Jeremy P., et al. "Quality protein intake is inversely related with abdominal fat." *Nutrition & metabolism* 9.1 (2012): 5.
[7] Weijs, Peter JM, and Robert R. Wolfe. "Exploration of the protein requirement during weight loss in obese older adults." *Clinical Nutrition* 35.2 (2016): 394-398.
[8] Marina, A. M., YB Che Man, and I. Amin. "Virgin coconut oil: emerging functional food oil." *Trends in Food Science & Technology* 20.10 (2009): 481-487.
[9] St-Onge, Marie-Pierre, and Aubrey Bosarge. "Weight-loss diet that includes consumption of medium-chain triacylglycerol oil leads to a greater rate of weight and fat mass loss than does olive oil." *The American journal of clinical nutrition* 87.3 (2008): 621-626.
[10] Radha Krishna, Y., et al. "Acute liver failure caused by 'fat burners' and dietary supplements: a case report and literature review." *Canadian Journal of Gastroenterology and Hepatology* 25.3 (2011): 157-160.

Chapter 6

[1] Jang, Meishiang, et al. "Cancer chemopreventive activity of resveratrol, a natural product derived from grapes." *Science* 275.5297 (1997): 218-220.
[2] Baur, Joseph A., et al. "Resveratrol improves health and survival of mice on a high-calorie diet." *Nature* 444.7117 (2006): 337-342.

[3] Timmers, Silvie, et al. "Calorie restriction-like effects of 30 days of resveratrol supplementation on energy metabolism and metabolic profile in obese humans." *Cell metabolism* 14.5 (2011): 612-622.

[4] Dolinsky, Vernon W., et al. "Improvements in skeletal muscle strength and cardiac function induced by resveratrol during exercise training contribute to enhanced exercise performance in rats." *The Journal of physiology* 590.11 (2012): 2783-2799.

[5] Juan, M. Emilia, et al. "trans-Resveratrol, a natural antioxidant from grapes, increases sperm output in healthy rats." *The Journal of nutrition* 135.4 (2005): 757-760.

[6] Stockinger, J., et al. "Caloric Restriction Mimetics Slow Aging of Neuromuscular Synapses and Muscle Fibers." *The journals of gerontology. Series A, Biological sciences and medical sciences* (2017).

[7] Diaz-Gerevini, Gustavo Tomas, et al. "Beneficial action of resveratrol: how and why?." *Nutrition* 32.2 (2016): 174-178.

[8] http://www.lifeextension.com/magazine/2007/3/report_resveratrol/page-04

[9] Pludowski, Pawel, et al. "Vitamin D effects on musculoskeletal health, immunity, autoimmunity, cardiovascular disease, cancer, fertility, pregnancy, dementia and mortality—a review of recent evidence." *Autoimmunity reviews* 12.10 (2013): 976-989.

[10] Lappe, Joan M., et al. "Vitamin D and calcium supplementation reduces cancer risk: results of a randomized trial." *The American journal of clinical nutrition* 85.6 (2007): 1586-1591.

[11] McDonnell, Sharon L., et al. "Serum 25-hydroxyvitamin D concentrations≥ 40 ng/mL are associated with> 65% lower cancer risk: pooled analysis of randomized trial and prospective cohort study." *PloS one* 11.4 (2016): e0152441.

[12] Giovannucci, Edward. "The epidemiology of vitamin D and cancer incidence and mortality: a review (United States)." *Cancer Causes & Control* 16.2 (2005): 83-95.

[13] Autier, Philippe, and Sara Gandini. "Vitamin D supplementation and total mortality: a meta-analysis of randomized controlled trials." *Archives of internal medicine* 167.16 (2007): 1730-1737.

[14] Anglin, Rebecca ES, et al. "Vitamin D deficiency and depression in adults: systematic review and meta-analysis." *The British journal of psychiatry* 202.2 (2013): 100-107.

[15] Jorde, R., et al. "Effects of vitamin D supplementation on symptoms of depression in overweight and obese subjects: randomized double blind trial." *Journal of internal medicine* 264.6 (2008): 599-609.

[16] Brøndum-Jacobsen, Peter, et al. "Skin cancer as a marker of sun exposure associates with myocardial infarction, hip fracture and death from any cause." *International journal of epidemiology* 42.5 (2013): 1486-1496.

[17] Lindqvist, P. G., et al. "Avoidance of sun exposure as a risk factor for major causes of death: a competing risk analysis of the Melanoma in Southern Sweden cohort." *Journal of internal medicine* 280.4 (2016): 375-387.

[18] Holick, Michael F., et al. "Evaluation, treatment, and prevention of vitamin D deficiency: an Endocrine Society clinical practice guideline." *The Journal of Clinical Endocrinology & Metabolism* 96.7 (2011): 1911-1930.

[19] Veugelers, Paul J., and John Paul Ekwaru. "A statistical error in the estimation of the recommended dietary allowance for vitamin D." *Nutrients* 6.10 (2014): 4472-4475.

[20] Nakachi, Kei, et al. "Preventive effects of drinking green tea on cancer and cardiovascular disease: epidemiological evidence for multiple targeting

prevention." *Biofactors* 13.1-4 (2000): 49-54.

[21] Ahmad, Nihal, et al. "Green tea constituent epigallocatechin-3-gallate and induction of apoptosis and cell cycle arrest in human carcinoma cells." *Journal of the National Cancer Institute* 89.24 (1997): 1881-1886.

[22] Xu, Yong, et al. "Inhibition of tobacco-specific nitrosamine-induced lung tumorigenesis in A/J mice by green tea and its major polyphenol as antioxidants." *Cancer Research* 52.14 (1992): 3875-3879.

[23] Bettuzzi, Saverio, et al. "Chemoprevention of human prostate cancer by oral administration of green tea catechins in volunteers with high-grade prostate intraepithelial neoplasia: a preliminary report from a one-year proof-of-principle study." *Cancer research* 66.2 (2006): 1234-1240.

[24] Shimizu, Masahito, et al. "Green tea extracts for the prevention of metachronous colorectal adenomas: a pilot study." *Cancer Epidemiology and Prevention Biomarkers* 17.11 (2008): 3020-3025.

[25] Roberts, Justin D., et al. "The effect of a decaffeinated green tea extract formula on fat oxidation, body composition and exercise performance." *Journal of the International Society of Sports Nutrition* 12.1 (2015): 1.

[26] Niu, Yucun, et al. "The phytochemical, EGCG, extends lifespan by reducing liver and kidney function damage and improving age-associated inflammation and oxidative stress in healthy rats." *Aging Cell* 12.6 (2013): 1041-1049.

[27] Mandel, Silvia A., et al. "Cell signaling pathways and iron chelation in the neurorestorative activity of green tea polyphenols: special reference to epigallocatechin gallate (EGCG)." *Journal of Alzheimer's disease* 15.2 (2008): 211-222.

[28] Weinreb, Orly, et al. "Neurological mechanisms of green tea polyphenols in Alzheimer's and Parkinson's diseases." *The Journal of nutritional biochemistry* 15.9 (2004): 506-516.

[29] Lambert, Joshua D., et al. "Hepatotoxicity of high oral dose (−)-epigallocatechin-3-gallate in mice." *Food and chemical toxicology* 48.1 (2010): 409-416.

[30] Weiss, David J., and Christopher R. Anderton. "Determination of catechins in matcha green tea by micellar electrokinetic chromatography." *Journal of Chromatography A* 1011.1 (2003): 173-180.

[31] Dong, Zigang, et al. "Inhibition of tumor promoter-induced activator protein 1 activation and cell transformation by tea polyphenols,(-)-epigallocatechin gallate, and theaflavins." *Cancer research* 57.19 (1997): 4414-4419.

[32] Miller, Nicholas J., et al. "The antioxidant properties of theaflavins and their gallate esters—radical scavengers or metal chelators?." *FEBS letters* 392.1 (1996): 40-44.

[33] Duffy, Stephen J., et al. "Short-and long-term black tea consumption reverses endothelial dysfunction in patients with coronary artery disease." *Circulation* 104.2 (2001): 151-156.

[34] Gardner, E. J., C. H. S. Ruxton, and A. R. Leeds. "Black tea—helpful or harmful? A review of the evidence." *European journal of clinical nutrition* 61.1 (2007): 3-18.

[35] Sesso, Howard D., et al. "Coffee and tea intake and the risk of myocardial infarction." *American Journal of Epidemiology* 149.2 (1999): 162-167.

[36] Yung, L. M., et al. "Tea polyphenols benefit vascular function." *Inflammopharmacology* 16.5 (2008): 230-234.

[37] Feng, L., et al. "TEA consumption reduces the incidence of neurocognitive disorders: Findings from the Singapore Longitudinal Aging Study." *The journal of nutrition, health & aging* 20.10 (2016): 1002-1009.

[38] Yin, Jun, Huili Xing, and Jianping Ye. "Efficacy of berberine in patients with type

2 diabetes mellitus." *Metabolism* 57.5 (2008): 712-717.

[39] Lee, Yun S., et al. "Berberine, a natural plant product, activates AMP-activated protein kinase with beneficial metabolic effects in diabetic and insulin-resistant states." *Diabetes* 55.8 (2006): 2256-2264.

[40] Yang, Jing, et al. "Berberine improves insulin sensitivity by inhibiting fat store and adjusting adipokines profile in human preadipocytes and metabolic syndrome patients." *Evidence-Based Complementary and Alternative Medicine* 2012 (2012).

[41] Fukuda, Kazunori, et al. "Inhibition by berberine of cyclooxygenase-2 transcriptional activity in human colon cancer cells." *Journal of ethnopharmacology* 66.2 (1999): 227-233.

[42] Kulkarni, Shrinivas K., and Ashish Dhir. "On the mechanism of antidepressant-like action of berberine chloride." *European Journal of Pharmacology* 589.1 (2008): 163-172.

[43] Kulkarni, S. K., and Ashish Dhir. "Berberine: a plant alkaloid with therapeutic potential for central nervous system disorders." *Phytotherapy Research* 24.3 (2010): 317-324.

[44] Dhillon, Navneet, et al. "Phase II trial of curcumin in patients with advanced pancreatic cancer." *Clinical Cancer Research* 14.14 (2008): 4491-4499.

[45] Jiao, Yan, et al. "Iron chelation in the biological activity of curcumin." *Free Radical Biology and Medicine* 40.7 (2006): 1152-1160.

[46] Anand, Preetha, et al. "Curcumin and cancer: an "old-age" disease with an "age-old" solution." *Cancer letters* 267.1 (2008): 133-164.

[47] Agrawal, Rahul, et al. "Effect of curcumin on brain insulin receptors and memory functions in STZ (ICV) induced dementia model of rat." *Pharmacological research* 61.3 (2010): 247-252.

[48] Begum, Aynun N., et al. "Curcumin structure-function, bioavailability, and efficacy in models of neuroinflammation and Alzheimer's disease." *Journal of Pharmacology and Experimental Therapeutics* 326.1 (2008): 196-208.

[49] Noratiqah, S. B., et al. "Natural Polyphenols in the Treatment of Alzheimer's Disease." *Current drug targets* (2017).

[50] B Mythri, R., and M. M Srinivas Bharath. "Curcumin: a potential neuroprotective agent in Parkinson's disease." *Current pharmaceutical design* 18.1 (2012): 91-99.

[51] Weisberg, Stuart P., Rudolph Leibel, and Drew V. Tortoriello. "Dietary curcumin significantly improves obesity-associated inflammation and diabetes in mouse models of diabesity." *Endocrinology* 149.7 (2008): 3549-3558.

[52] Chandran, Binu, and Ajay Goel. "A randomized, pilot study to assess the efficacy and safety of curcumin in patients with active rheumatoid arthritis." *Phytotherapy research* 26.11 (2012): 1719-1725.

[53] Hanai, Hiroyuki, et al. "Curcumin maintenance therapy for ulcerative colitis: randomized, multicenter, double-blind, placebo-controlled trial." *Clinical Gastroenterology and Hepatology* 4.12 (2006): 1502-1506.

[54] Kulkarni, S. K., Ashish Dhir, and Kiran Kumar Akula. "Potentials of curcumin as an antidepressant." *The Scientific World Journal* 9 (2009): 1233-1241.

[55] Wang, Long. "Curcumin prevents the non-alcoholic fatty hepatitis via mitochondria protection and apoptosis reduction." *International journal of clinical and experimental pathology* 8.9 (2015): 11503.

[56] Chainani-Wu, Nita. "Safety and anti-inflammatory activity of curcumin: a component of tumeric (Curcuma longa)." *The Journal of Alternative & Complementary Medicine* 9.1 (2003): 161-168.

[57] Shamsuddin, Abulkalam M., Ivana Vucenik, and Katharine E. Cole. "IP6: a novel anti-cancer agent." *Life sciences* 61.4 (1997): 343-354.

[58] Somasundar, Ponnandai, et al. "Inositol hexaphosphate (IP6): A novel treatment for pancreatic cancer 1." *Journal of Surgical Research* 126.2 (2005): 199-203.

[59] Mounsey, Ross B., and Peter Teismann. "Chelators in the treatment of iron accumulation in Parkinson's disease." *International journal of cell biology* 2012 (2012).

[60] Anekonda, Thimmappa S., et al. "Phytic acid as a potential treatment for alzheimer's pathology: evidence from animal and in vitro models." *Journal of Alzheimer's Disease* 23.1 (2011): 21-35.

[61] Bhowmik, Anwesha, et al. "Inositol hexa phosphoric acid (phytic acid), a nutraceuticals, attenuates iron-induced oxidative stress and alleviates liver injury in iron overloaded mice." *Biomedicine & Pharmacotherapy* 87 (2017): 443-450.

[62] Grases, F. E. L. I. X., and A. N. T. O. N. I. A. Costa-Bauza. "Phytate (IP6) is a powerful agent on preventing calcification in biological fluids. Usefulness in renal lithiasis treatment." *Anticancer research* 19.5 (1999): 3717-3722.

[63] Vucenik, Ivana, and AbulKalam M. Shamsuddin. "Cancer inhibition by inositol hexaphosphate (IP6) and inositol: from laboratory to clinic." *The Journal of nutrition* 133.11 (2003): 3778S-3784S.

[64] Schrauzer, Gerhard N. "Lithium: occurrence, dietary intakes, nutritional essentiality." *Journal of the American College of Nutrition* 21.1 (2002): 14-21.

[65] Sugawara, Norio, et al. "Lithium in tap water and suicide mortality in Japan." *International journal of environmental research and public health* 10.11 (2013): 6044-6048.

[66] Zarse, Kim, et al. "Low-dose lithium uptake promotes longevity in humans and metazoans." *European journal of nutrition* 50.5 (2011): 387-389.

[67] Fornai, Francesco, et al. "Lithium delays progression of amyotrophic lateral sclerosis." *Proceedings of the National Academy of Sciences* 105.6 (2008): 2052-2057.

[68] Calonge, Ned, et al. "Aspirin for the prevention of cardiovascular disease." *Annals of internal medicine* 150.6 (2009): 396-404.

[69] Thun, Michael J., et al. "Aspirin use and risk of fatal cancer." *Cancer research* 53.6 (1993): 1322-1327.

[70] Rothwell, Peter M., et al. "Effect of daily aspirin on long-term risk of death due to cancer: analysis of individual patient data from randomised trials." *The Lancet* 377.9759 (2011): 31-41.

[71] http://www.nytimes.com/2012/03/21/health/research/studies-link-aspirin-daily-use-to-reduced-cancer-risk.html

[72] Cuzick, Jack, et al. "Estimates of benefits and harms of prophylactic use of aspirin in the general population." *Annals of Oncology* (2014): mdu225.

[73] Lapi, F., et al. "Risk of prostate cancer in low-dose aspirin users: A retrospective cohort study." *International journal of cancer* 139.1 (2016): 205-211.

[74] Rothwell, Peter M., et al. "Effect of daily aspirin on risk of cancer metastasis: a study of incident cancers during randomised controlled trials." *The Lancet* 379.9826 (2012): 1591-1601.

[75] Ralph, Stephen John, et al. "Hitting the Bull's-Eye in Metastatic Cancers—NSAIDs Elevate ROS in Mitochondria, Inducing Malignant Cell Death." *Pharmaceuticals* 8.1 (2015): 62-106.

[76] Cuzick, Jack, et al. "Estimates of benefits and harms of prophylactic use of aspirin in the general population." *Annals of Oncology* (2014): mdu225.

[77] Agus, David B., et al. "The Long-Term Benefits of Increased Aspirin Use by At-

Risk Americans Aged 50 and Older." *PloS one* 11.11 (2016): e0166103.

Shmerling, Robert, "Is aspirin a wonder drug?"
http://www.health.harvard.edu/blog/aspirin-wonder-drug-2016122210916

[78] Strong, Randy, et al. "Nordihydroguaiaretic acid and aspirin increase lifespan of genetically heterogeneous male mice." *Aging cell* 7.5 (2008): 641-650.

[79] Lutchman, Vicky, et al. "Discovery of plant extracts that greatly delay yeast chronological aging and have different effects on longevity-defining cellular processes." *Oncotarget* 7.13 (2016): 16542.

[80] Hawthorne, A. B., et al. "Aspirin-induced gastric mucosal damage: prevention by enteric-coating and relation to prostaglandin synthesis." *British journal of clinical pharmacology* 32.1 (1991): 77-83.

[81] Geleijnse, Johanna M., et al. "Dietary intake of menaquinone is associated with a reduced risk of coronary heart disease: the Rotterdam Study." *The Journal of nutrition* 134.11 (2004): 3100-3105.

[82] Gast, Gerrie-Cor M., et al. "A high menaquinone intake reduces the incidence of coronary heart disease." *Nutrition, Metabolism and Cardiovascular Diseases* 19.7 (2009): 504-510.

[83] Nimptsch, Katharina, et al. "Dietary vitamin K intake in relation to cancer incidence and mortality: results from the Heidelberg cohort of the European Prospective Investigation into Cancer and Nutrition (EPIC-Heidelberg)." *The American journal of clinical nutrition* (2010): ajcn-28691.

[84] Bell, Griffith A., et al. "Use of glucosamine and chondroitin in relation to mortality." *European journal of epidemiology* 27.8 (2012): 593-603.

[85] Weimer, Sandra, et al. "D-Glucosamine supplementation extends life span of nematodes and of ageing mice." *Nature communications* 5 (2014).

[86] Caramés, Beatriz, et al. "Glucosamine activates autophagy in vitro and in vivo." *Arthritis & Rheumatism* 65.7 (2013): 1843-1852.

[87] Hou, Yongqing, Yulong Yin, and Guoyao Wu. "Dietary essentiality of "nutritionally non-essential amino acids" for animals and humans." *Experimental Biology and Medicine* 240.8 (2015): 997-1007.

[88] Sanz, Alberto, et al. "Methionine restriction decreases mitochondrial oxygen radical generation and leak as well as oxidative damage to mitochondrial DNA and proteins." *The FASEB Journal* 20.8 (2006): 1064-1073.

[89] Sekhar, Rajagopal V., et al. "Deficient synthesis of glutathione underlies oxidative stress in aging and can be corrected by dietary cysteine and glycine supplementation." *The American journal of clinical nutrition* 94.3 (2011): 847-853.

[90] Yamadera, Wataru, et al. "Glycine ingestion improves subjective sleep quality in human volunteers, correlating with polysomnographic changes." *Sleep and Biological Rhythms* 5.2 (2007): 126-131.

[91] Anisimov, Vladimir N., et al. "Dose-dependent effect of melatonin on life span and spontaneous tumor incidence in female SHR mice." *Experimental gerontology* 38.4 (2003): 449-461.

[92] Lemoine, Patrick, et al. "Prolonged-release melatonin improves sleep quality and morning alertness in insomnia patients aged 55 years and older and has no withdrawal effects." *Journal of sleep research* 16.4 (2007): 372-380.

[93] Buscemi, Nina, et al. "The efficacy and safety of exogenous melatonin for primary sleep disorders." *Journal of general internal medicine* 20.12 (2005): 1151-1158.

[94] https://sleep.org/articles/how-much-melatonin-to-take/

[95] Zhu, Yi, et al. "The Achilles' heel of senescent cells: from transcriptome to senolytic drugs." *Aging cell* 14.4 (2015): 644-658.

[96] Russo, Maria, et al. "The flavonoid quercetin in disease prevention and therapy:

facts and fancies." *Biochemical pharmacology* 83.1 (2012): 6-15.

[97] Jones, Eleri, and R. E. Hughes. "Quercetin, flavonoids and the life-span of mice." *Experimental Gerontology* 17.3 (1982): 213-217.

Spindler, Stephen R., et al. "Influence on longevity of blueberry, cinnamon, green and black tea, pomegranate, sesame, curcumin, morin, pycnogenol, quercetin, and taxifolin fed iso-calorically to long-lived, F1 hybrid mice." *Rejuvenation Research* 16.2 (2013): 143-151.

[98] Baar, M. et al., "Targeted Apoptosis of Senescent Cells Restores Tissue Homeostasis in Response to Chemotoxicity and Aging". *Cell*, Volume 169, Issue 1, p132–147.e16, (2017)

[99] Dröge, Wulf. "Oxidative stress and ageing: is ageing a cysteine deficiency syndrome?." *Philosophical Transactions of the Royal Society of London B: Biological Sciences* 360.1464 (2005): 2355-2372.

[100] Morris, Gerwyn, et al. "The glutathione system: a new drug target in neuroimmune disorders." *Molecular neurobiology* 50.3 (2014): 1059-1084.

[101] Berk, Michael, et al. "The efficacy of N-acetylcysteine as an adjunctive treatment in bipolar depression: an open label trial." *Journal of affective disorders* 135.1 (2011): 389-394.

[102] Berk, Michael, et al. "The promise of N-acetylcysteine in neuropsychiatry." *Trends in pharmacological sciences* 34.3 (2013): 167-177.

[103] Maes, Michael, et al. "Increased 8-hydroxy-deoxyguanosine, a marker of oxidative damage to DNA, in major depression and myalgic encephalomyelitis/chronic fatigue syndrome." *Neuroendocrinology Letters* 30.6 (2009): 715.

[104] Bounous, G., and J. Molson. "Competition for glutathione precursors between the immune system and the skeletal muscle: pathogenesis of chronic fatigue syndrome." *Medical hypotheses* 53.4 (1999): 347-349.

[105] Morris, Gerwyn, et al. "The glutathione system: a new drug target in neuroimmune disorders." *Molecular neurobiology* 50.3 (2014): 1059-1084.

[106] Maes, Michael, and Jean-Claude Leunis. "Normalization of leaky gut in chronic fatigue syndrome (CFS) is accompanied by a clinical improvement: effects of age, duration of illness and the translocation of LPS from gram-negative bacteria." *Neuroendocrinology Letters* 29.6 (2008): 902.

[107] De Flora, S., C. Grassi, and L. Carati. "Attenuation of influenza-like symptomatology and improvement of cell-mediated immunity with long-term N-acetylcysteine treatment." *European Respiratory Journal* 10.7 (1997): 1535-1541.

[108] Rasmussen, J. B., and C. Glennow. "Reduction in days of illness after long-term treatment with N-acetylcysteine controlled-release tablets in patients with chronic bronchitis." *European Respiratory Journal* 1.4 (1988): 351-355.

[109] Ballatori, Nazzareno, Michael W. Lieberman, and Wei Wang. "N-acetylcysteine as an antidote in methylmercury poisoning." *Environmental health perspectives* 106.5 (1998): 267.

Ottenwälder, H., and P. Simon. "Differential effect of N-acetylcysteine on excretion of the metals Hg, Cd, Pb and Au." *Archives of toxicology* 60.5 (1987): 401-402.

[110] Corn, Sarah D., and Thomas J. Barstow. "Effects of oral N-acetylcysteine on fatigue, critical power, and W′ in exercising humans." *Respiratory physiology & neurobiology* 178.2 (2011): 261-268.

[111] Kelly, Megan K., et al. "Effects of N-acetylcysteine on respiratory muscle fatigue during heavy exercise." *Respiratory physiology & neurobiology* 165.1 (2009): 67-72.

[112] Trewin, Adam J., et al. "N-acetylcysteine alters substrate metabolism during

high-intensity cycle exercise in well-trained humans." *Applied Physiology, Nutrition, and Metabolism* 38.12 (2013): 1217-1227.

[113] Dröge, Wulf. "Oxidative stress and ageing: is ageing a cysteine deficiency syndrome?." *Philosophical Transactions of the Royal Society of London B: Biological Sciences* 360.1464 (2005): 2355-2372.

[114] Hauer, Klaus, et al. "Improvement in muscular performance and decrease in tumor necrosis factor level in old age after antioxidant treatment." *Journal of molecular medicine* 81.2 (2003): 118-125.

[115] Mercola, Joseph; "N-acetylcysteine (NAC): This Common Antioxidant Supplement Could Cause You Loads of Trouble" http://articles.mercola.com/sites/articles/archive/2007/09/25/this-common-antioxidant-supplement-could-cause-you-loads-of-trouble.aspx Retrieved April 10, 2017.

[116] Frank Giorlando MBBS, BMedSc. "N-acetylcysteine in psychiatry: current therapeutic evidence and potential mechanisms of action." *Journal of psychiatry & neuroscience: JPN* 36.2 (2011): 78.

[117] Goepp, Julius, M.D.: The Overlooked Compound That Saves Lives. http://www.lifeextension.com/Magazine/2010/5/N-Acetyl-Cysteine/Page-01. Retrieved April 10, 2017

[118] Atkuri, Kondala R., et al. "N-Acetylcysteine—a safe antidote for cysteine/glutathione deficiency." *Current opinion in pharmacology* 7.4 (2007): 355-359.

[119] Zarse, Kim, Saskia Jabin, and Michael Ristow. "L-Theanine extends lifespan of adult Caenorhabditis elegans." *European Journal of Nutrition* 51.6 (2012): 765-768.

[120] Juneja, Lekh Raj, et al. "L-theanine—a unique amino acid of green tea and its relaxation effect in humans." *Trends in Food Science & Technology* 10.6 (1999): 199-204.

[121] Ritsner, Michael S., et al. "L-theanine relieves positive, activation, and anxiety symptoms in patients with schizophrenia and schizoaffective disorder: an 8-week, randomized, double-blind, placebo-controlled, 2-center study." *Journal of Clinical Psychiatry* 72.1 (2011): 34.

[122] Borzelleca, J. F., D. Peters, and W. Hall. "A 13-week dietary toxicity and toxicokinetic study with L-theanine in rats." *Food and chemical toxicology* 44.7 (2006): 1158-1166.

[123] https://www.drugs.com/npp/l-theanine.html

[124] Keenan, Emma K., et al. "How much theanine in a cup of tea? Effects of tea type and method of preparation." *Food chemistry* 125.2 (2011): 588-594.

[125] Pinckaers, Philippe JM, et al. "Ketone Bodies and Exercise Performance: The Next Magic Bullet or Merely Hype?." *Sports Medicine* (2016): 1-9.

[126] Veech, Richard L., et al. "Ketone bodies mimic the life span extending properties of caloric restriction." *IUBMB life* (2017).

[127] Tresserra-Rimbau, Anna, et al. "Polyphenol intake and mortality risk: a re-analysis of the PREDIMED trial." *BMC medicine* 12.1 (2014): 77.

[128] Tresserra-Rimbau, Anna, et al. "Inverse association between habitual polyphenol intake and incidence of cardiovascular events in the PREDIMED study." *Nutrition, Metabolism and Cardiovascular Diseases* 24.6 (2014): 639-647.

[129] Pérez-Jiménez, J., et al. "Identification of the 100 richest dietary sources of polyphenols: an application of the Phenol-Explorer database." *European journal of clinical nutrition* 64 (2010): S112-S120.

[130] http://www.businessinsider.com/ray-kurzweils-immortality-diet-2015-4

https://www.quora.com/Which-150-supplements-does-Ray-Kurzweil-take-daily
[131] Ravnskov, Uffe, et al. "Lack of an association or an inverse association between low-density-lipoprotein cholesterol and mortality in the elderly: a systematic review." *BMJ open* 6.6 (2016): e010401.
[132] Engelberg, Hyman. "Low serum cholesterol and suicide." *The Lancet* 339.8795 (1992): 727-729.

Chapter 7

[1] https://www.aad.org/public/diseases/acne-and-rosacea/acne
[2] Cordain, Loren, et al. "Acne vulgaris: a disease of Western civilization." *Archives of dermatology* 138.12 (2002): 1584-1590.
[3] Lindeberg, Staffan, et al. "Low serum insulin in traditional Pacific Islanders—the Kitava Study." *Metabolism* 48.10 (1999): 1216-1219.
[4] https://www.drugs.com/sfx/accutane-side-effects.html
[5] Patel, Mital, et al. "The development of antimicrobial resistance due to the antibiotic treatment of acne vulgaris: a review." *Journal of drugs in dermatology: JDD* 9.6 (2010): 655-664.
[6] Sagransky, Matt, Brad A. Yentzer, and Steven R. Feldman. "Benzoyl peroxide: a review of its current use in the treatment of acne vulgaris." *Expert opinion on pharmacotherapy* 10.15 (2009): 2555-2562.
[7] Bowe, Whitney P., and Alan R. Shalita. "Effective over-the-counter acne treatments." *Seminars in cutaneous medicine and surgery*. Vol. 27. No. 3. Frontline Medical Communications, 2008.
[8] Sahni, Sumit, et al. "The use of iron chelators in biocidal compositions: evaluation of patent, WO2014059417A1." *Expert opinion on therapeutic patents* 25.3 (2015): 367-372.
[9] Pourzand, Charareh, et al. "Ultraviolet A radiation induces immediate release of iron in human primary skin fibroblasts: the role of ferritin." *Proceedings of the National Academy of Sciences* 96.12 (1999): 6751-6756.
[10] Bissett, Donald L., and James F. McBride. "Iron content of human epidermis from sun-exposed and non-exposed body sites." *JOURNAL-SOCIETY OF COSMETIC CHEMISTS* 43 (1992): 215-215.
[11] Bissett, Donald L., Ranjit Chatterjee, and Daniel P. Hannon. "Chronic Ultraviolet Radiation-Induced Increase In Skin Iron And The Photoprotective Effect Of Topically Applied Iron Chelators 1." *Photochemistry and Photobiology* 54.2 (1991): 215-223.
[12] Mitani, Hiroaki, et al. "Prevention of the photodamage in the hairless mouse dorsal skin by kojic acid as an iron chelator." *European journal of pharmacology* 411.1 (2001): 169-174.
[13] Bissett, Donald L., John E. Oblong, and Cynthia A. Berge. "Niacinamide: AB vitamin that improves aging facial skin appearance." *Dermatologic surgery* 31.s1 (2005): 860-866.
[14] Zhoh, Choon-Koo, et al. "The effects of inositol extracted from rice on the skin." *Journal of the Society of Cosmetic Scientists of Korea* 27.1 (2001): 83-98.
[15] Piérard-Franchimont, C., et al. "Ketoconazole shampoo: effect of long-term use in androgenic alopecia." *Dermatology* 196.4 (1998): 474-477.
[16] Matilainen, Veikko, Pentti Koskela, and Sirkka Keinänen-Kiukaanniemi. "Early androgenetic alopecia as a marker of insulin resistance." *The Lancet* 356.9236 (2000): 1165-1166.
[17] Ford, Earl S., David S. Freedman, and Tim Byers. "Baldness and ischemic heart

disease in a national sample of men." *American journal of epidemiology* 143.7 (1996).

[18] DeAngelis, Yvonne M., et al. "Three etiologic facets of dandruff and seborrheic dermatitis: Malassezia fungi, sebaceous lipids, and individual sensitivity." *Journal of Investigative Dermatology Symposium Proceedings*. Vol. 10. No. 3. Elsevier, 2005.

[19] Squire, R. A., and K. Goode. "A randomised, single-blind, single-centre clinical trial to evaluate comparative clinical efficacy of shampoos containing ciclopirox olamine (1.5%) and salicylic acid (3%), or ketoconazole (2%, Nizoral®) for the treatment of dandruff/seborrhoeic dermatitis." *Journal of dermatological treatment* 13.2 (2002): 51-60.

[20] Panahi, Y., et al. "Rosemary oil vs minoxidil 2% for the treatment of androgenetic alopecia: a randomized comparative trial." *Skinmed* 13.1 (2014): 15-21.

[21] Baratta, M. Tiziana, et al. "Chemical composition, antimicrobial and antioxidative activity of laurel, sage, rosemary, oregano and coriander essential oils." *Journal of Essential Oil Research* 10.6 (1998): 618-627.

Chapter 8

[1] Rehm, Jürgen, et al. "Alcohol-related morbidity and mortality." *Alcohol Res. Health* 140 (2003): C00-C97.

[2] Di Castelnuovo, Augusto, et al. "Alcohol dosing and total mortality in men and women: an updated meta-analysis of 34 prospective studies." *Archives of Internal Medicine* 166.22 (2006): 2437-2445.

[3] Kanazawa, Satoshi, and Josephine EEU Hellberg. "Intelligence and substance use." *Review of general psychology* 14.4 (2010): 382.

[4] Gottfredson, Linda S., and Ian J. Deary. "Intelligence predicts health and longevity, but why?." *Current Directions in Psychological Science* 13.1 (2004): 1-4.

[5] Gronbaek, Morten, et al. "Mortality associated with moderate intakes of wine, beer, or spirits." *Bmj* 310.6988 (1995): 1165-1169.

[6] Trichopoulou, Antonia, Christina Bamia, and Dimitrios Trichopoulos. "Anatomy of health effects of Mediterranean diet: Greek EPIC prospective cohort study." *Bmj* 338 (2009): b2337.

[7] Vinson, Joe A., Karolyn Teufel, and Nancy Wu. "Red wine, dealcoholized red wine, and especially grape juice, inhibit atherosclerosis in a hamster model." *Atherosclerosis* 156.1 (2001): 67-72.

[8] Carmelli, Dorit, et al. "World War II-veteran male twins who are discordant for alcohol consumption: 24-year mortality." *American Journal of Public Health* 85.1 (1995): 99-101.

[9] Wannamethee, S. Goya, and A. Gerald Shaper. "Lifelong teetotallers, ex-drinkers and drinkers: mortality and the incidence of major coronary heart disease events in middle-aged British men." *International Journal of Epidemiology* 26.3 (1997): 523-531.

[10] Foster, David A. "Reduced mortality and moderate alcohol consumption: the phospholipase D-mTOR connection." *Cell Cycle* 9.7 (2010): 1291-1294.

[11] Doll, Richard, et al. "Mortality in relation to consumption of alcohol: 13 years' observations on male British doctors." *BMJ: British Medical Journal* 309.6959 (1994): 911.

[12] Lelbach, Werner K. "Cirrhosis in the alcoholic and its relation to the volume of alcohol abuse." *Annals of the New York Academy of Sciences* 252.1 (1975): 85-105.

[13] Nanji, Amin A., Charles L. Mendenhall, and Samuel W. French. "Beef fat prevents

alcoholic liver disease in the rat." *Alcoholism: Clinical and Experimental Research* 13.1 (1989): 15-19.

[14] Nanji, Amin A., et al. "Dietary saturated fatty acids down-regulate cyclooxygenase-2 and tumor necrosis factor alfa and reverse fibrosis in alcohol-induced liver disease in the rat." *Hepatology* 26.6 (1997): 1538-1545.

[15] Corrao, Giovanni, et al. "A meta-analysis of alcohol consumption and the risk of 15 diseases." *Preventive Medicine* 38.5 (2004): 613-619.

[16] Maheswaran, Ravi, et al. "High blood pressure due to alcohol. A rapidly reversible effect." *Hypertension* 17.6 Pt 1 (1991): 787-792.

[17] Gruchow, Harvey W., et al. "Alcohol consumption, nutrient intake and relative body weight among US adults." *The American journal of clinical nutrition* 42.2 (1985): 289-295.

Chapter 9

[1] Bischoff-Ferrari, Heike A., et al. "Calcium intake and hip fracture risk in men and women: a meta-analysis of prospective cohort studies and randomized controlled trials." *The American journal of clinical nutrition* 86.6 (2007): 1780-1790.

[2] Joshi, Parag H., et al. "Coronary artery Calcium predicts Cardiovascular events in participants with a low lifetime risk of Cardiovascular disease: the Multi-Ethnic Study of Atherosclerosis (MESA)." *Atherosclerosis* 246 (2016): 367-373.

[3] Bolland, Mark J., et al. "Effect of calcium supplements on risk of myocardial infarction and cardiovascular events: meta-analysis." *BMJ* 341 (2010): c3691.

[4] Li, Kuanrong, et al. "Associations of dietary calcium intake and calcium supplementation with myocardial infarction and stroke risk and overall cardiovascular mortality in the Heidelberg cohort of the European Prospective Investigation into Cancer and Nutrition study (EPIC-Heidelberg)." *Heart* 98.12 (2012): 920-925.

[5] Michaëlsson, Karl, et al. "Long term calcium intake and rates of all cause and cardiovascular mortality: community based prospective longitudinal cohort study." *Bmj* 346 (2013): f228.

[6] Elwood, P. C., et al. "Milk consumption, stroke, and heart attack risk: evidence from the Caerphilly cohort of older men." *Journal of epidemiology and community health* 59.6 (2005): 502-505.

[7] Nimptsch, Katharina, et al. "Dietary vitamin K intake in relation to cancer incidence and mortality: results from the Heidelberg cohort of the European Prospective Investigation into Cancer and Nutrition (EPIC-Heidelberg)." *The American journal of clinical nutrition* (2010): ajcn-28691.

[8] P.D. Mangan. *Dumping Iron: How to Ditch This Secret Killer and Reclaim Your Health*. Phalanx Press, 2016

[9] Kent, Susan, Eugene D. Weinberg, and Patricia Stuart-Macadam. "Dietary and prophylactic iron supplements." *Human Nature* 1.1 (1990): 53-79.

[10] Wu, Tiejian, et al. "Serum iron, copper and zinc concentrations and risk of cancer mortality in US adults." *Annals of epidemiology* 14.3 (2004): 195-201.

[11] Brewer, George J. "Risks of copper and iron toxicity during aging in humans." *Chemical research in toxicology* 23.2 (2009): 319-326.

[12] Matos, Liliana, Alexandra Gouveia, and Henrique Almeida. "Copper ability to induce premature senescence in human fibroblasts." *Age* 34.4 (2012): 783-794.

[13] Ristow, Michael, et al. "Antioxidants prevent health-promoting effects of physical exercise in humans." *Proceedings of the National Academy of Sciences* 106.21 (2009): 8665-8670.

[14] Bjelakovic, Goran, et al. "Mortality in randomized trials of antioxidant supplements for primary and secondary prevention: systematic review and meta-analysis." *Jama* 297.8 (2007): 842-857.

[15] Underwood, Benjamin R., et al. "Antioxidants can inhibit basal autophagy and enhance neurodegeneration in models of polyglutamine disease." *Human molecular genetics* 19.17 (2010): 3413-3429.

[16] Johnston, Carol S., Gillean M. Barkyoumb, and Sara S. Schumacher. "Vitamin C supplementation slightly improves physical activity levels and reduces cold incidence in men with marginal vitamin C status: A randomized controlled trial." *Nutrients* 6.7 (2014): 2572-2583.

[17] Hemilä, Harri. "Vitamin C and Infections." *Nutrients* 9.4 (2017): 339.

[18] Zhang, Michelle, et al. "Vitamin C provision improves mood in acutely hospitalized patients." *Nutrition* 27.5 (2011): 530-533.

[19] Marik, Paul E., et al. "Hydrocortisone, Vitamin C and Thiamine for the Treatment of Severe Sepsis and Septic Shock: A Retrospective Before-After Study." *CHEST Journal* (2016).

[20] Evans, W., et al. "Ostarine increases lean body mass and improves physical performance in healthy elderly subjects: implications for cancer cachexia patients." *Journal of Clinical Oncology* 25.90180 (2007): 9119-9119.

[21] http://fluoridealert.org/issues/health/brain/

[22] http://fluoridealert.org/issues/health/fertility/

Chapter 10

[1] http://articles.latimes.com/2011/sep/17/local/la-me-drugs-epidemic-20110918

[2] Hayward, Rodney A., and Timothy P. Hofer. "Estimating hospital deaths due to medical errors: preventability is in the eye of the reviewer." *Jama* 286.4 (2001): 415-420.

[3] Leape, Lucian L. "Institute of Medicine medical error figures are not exaggerated." *Jama* 284.1 (2000): 95-97.

[4] https://www.cdc.gov/hai/surveillance/

[5] Gøtzsche, Peter C., Allan H. Young, and John Crace. "Maudsley Debate: Does long term use of psychiatric drugs cause more harm than good?." *The BMJ* 350 (2015).

[6] Kripke, Daniel F., Robert D. Langer, and Lawrence E. Kline. "Hypnotics' association with mortality or cancer: a matched cohort study." *BMJ open* 2.1 (2012): e000850.

[7] https://www.drugabuse.gov/publications/drugfacts/drug-related-hospital-emergency-room-visits

[8] http://articles.mercola.com/sites/articles/archive/2016/02/10/5-reasons-why-you-should-not-take-statins.aspx

[9] Okuyama, Harumi, et al. "Statins stimulate atherosclerosis and heart failure: pharmacological mechanisms." *Expert review of clinical pharmacology* 8.2 (2015): 189-199.

[10] Golomb, Beatrice A., et al. "Statin effects on aggression: results from the UCSD Statin Study, a randomized control trial." *PloS one* 10.7 (2015): e0124451.

[11] http://www.orthomolecular.org/resources/omns/v13n02.shtml

[12] https://www.statista.com/statistics/261303/total-number-of-retail-prescriptions-filled-annually-in-the-us/

[13] https://www.statista.com/statistics/263102/pharmaceutical-market-worldwide-revenue-since-2001/

[1] Welsh, Jean A., et al. "Consumption of added sugars is decreasing in the United

States." *The American journal of clinical nutrition* 94.3 (2011): 726-734.

[2] Yang, Quanhe, et al. "Added sugar intake and cardiovascular diseases mortality among US adults." *JAMA Internal Medicine* 174.4 (2014): 516-524.

[3] DiNicolantonio, James J., and Sean C. Lucan. "The wrong white crystals: not salt but sugar as aetiological in hypertension and cardiometabolic disease." *Open Heart* 1.1 (2014): e000167.

[4] Basciano, Heather, Lisa Federico, and Khosrow Adeli. "Fructose, insulin resistance, and metabolic dyslipidemia." *Nutrition & metabolism* 2.1 (2005): 5.

[5] Bray, George A., Samara Joy Nielsen, and Barry M. Popkin. "Consumption of high-fructose corn syrup in beverages may play a role in the epidemic of obesity." *The American journal of clinical nutrition* 79.4 (2004): 537-543.

[6] Liu, Simin, et al. "A prospective study of dietary glycemic load, carbohydrate intake, and risk of coronary heart disease in US women." *The American Journal of Clinical Nutrition* 71.6 (2000): 1455-1461.

[7] Thorogood, Adrian, et al. "Isolated aerobic exercise and weight loss: a systematic review and meta-analysis of randomized controlled trials." *The American journal of medicine* 124.8 (2011): 747-755.

Made in the USA
Monee, IL
12 January 2021